Saltwater Cure

Saltwater Cure

TRUE STORIES OF THE
TRANSFORMATIVE POWER
OF THE OCEAN

Ali Gripper

murdoch books

Sydney | London

Published in 2024 by Murdoch Books, an imprint of Allen & Unwin

Excerpts on pp. 5, 7, 9, 13 and 18 from *Beneath the Waves* © Layne Beachley & Michael Gordon 2009; pp. 49–52 and 55 from *Valerie Taylor: An Adventurous Life* © Valerie Taylor with Ben Mckelvey 2021

Murdoch Books Australia
Cammeraygal Country
83 Alexander Street, Crows Nest NSW 2065
Phone: +61 (0)2 8425 0100
murdochbooks.com.au
info@murdochbooks.com.au

Murdoch Books UK
Ormond House, 26–27 Boswell Street, London WC1N 3JZ
Phone: +44 (0) 20 8785 5995
murdochbooks.co.uk
info@murdochbooks.co.uk

A catalogue record for this book is available from the National Library of Australia

ISBN 978 1 76150 000 8

Cover and text design by Sarah Odgers
Typeset by Midland Typesetters
Printed and bound in Great Britain by CPI Group (UK) Ltd, Croydon, CR0 4YY

DISCLAIMER: The content presented in this book is meant for inspiration and informational purposes only. The author and publisher claim no responsibility to any person or entity for any liability, loss, or damage caused or alleged to be caused directly or indirectly as a result of the use, application, or interpretation of the material in this book.

Every reasonable effort has been made to trace the owners of copyright materials in this book, but in some instances this has proven impossible. The author(s) and publisher will be glad to receive information leading to more complete acknowledgements in subsequent printings of the book and in the meantime extend their apologies for any omissions.

Murdoch Books acknowledges the Traditional Owners of the Country on which we live and work. We pay our respects to all Aboriginal and Torres Strait Islander Elders, past and present.

10 9 8 7 6 5 4 3 2 1

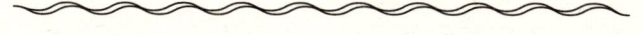

For my parents, Jillian and Terry,
two great Australians.
And for marine life everywhere.

This book was written on land first inhabited by the Gadigal and Bidjigal people. I pay my respects to these traditional custodians and their deep connection to the land and sea around us. I thank them for protecting this coastline and its ecosystems for more than 60,000 years.

Contents

Introduction

~~~

I GREW UP in the western suburbs of Sydney, and it was always a highlight when we would stash our foam surfboards in the back of the Holden Kingswood on the weekend and drive to the beach at Maroubra or Coogee, near my grandparents' home. I savoured every moment: the north-easterly breeze and the thrill of catching a big bottle-green wave back to the shore on my father's shoulders.

Today, I am still uplifted every time I catch sight of the horizon from the coast – all that sea, and the possibility of spotting a pod of dolphins or, if I visit at the right time of year, the arched black back of a humpback whale.

Plunging under the surface, even in the winter months – in my wetsuit when the water temperature drops to 14 degrees Celsius – and being enveloped in foam and whitewash never fails to put me in a positive frame of mind.

Saltwater Cure first came into being after I interviewed Valerie Taylor for *The Sydney Morning Herald* about a shark exhibition at the Australian Museum. The grande dame of underwater cinematography seemed lit from within as she sat chatting on her sofa. Valerie is in her late 80s now, but she is still snorkelling; she says being underwater makes her feel as if she's about 40 years old again.

I was astonished by the way the ocean had so dramatically changed the course of her life, from that of a spearfisher to a fierce conservationist, a woman dedicated to eradicating shark nets from Australia.

Her story would not let me go, and I began wondering if the ocean could have the same transformative qualities for anyone who came into contact with it. What was this mysterious elixir that could make people feel young again, that could heal, that could soothe and change an entire perspective on life?

One thing quickly became clear as I launched into the interviews: not only did the power of the ocean transcend age, faith, gender, cultural background and physical ability, it imbued every person I spoke to with a great respect for mother nature. Whether they were swimming, surfing, sailing, diving, fishing or walking along the shoreline, they all mentioned that they were yielding to something greater than themselves, something they could not control or change.

The more time people spend in the salt water, it seems, the more they care about it. Many were deeply concerned by the stresses to which the ocean has been subjected due to climate change, a rising thermostat and the increase in ocean refuse.

In return, the ocean gives back to them in abundant ways.

It has given blind marathon swimmer James Pittar the freedom to compete with able-bodied athletes for the first time in his life. On land he is held back by his disability, but in the ocean he can move wherever he likes, at whatever speed he likes, without bumping into anything or anyone.

For children on the autism spectrum, the sense of being held by the salt water – with a surf lifesaver on either side of them – gives them a feeling of being at peace.

It was a privilege to spend time with around-the-world sailor Jessica Watson and learn how being out on the ocean helped her find sparks of joy again after her world turned dark, grappling with the grief of losing her partner.

And I have nothing but admiration for world-champion surfer Layne Beachley and the way proving herself over and over again out in the deep gave her a sense of love and approval when she was struggling to come to terms with the fact that she was adopted.

I was moved by all of these stories, including the one from migrants Rajbir Kaur and Sumit Singh, who learned to swim later in life and now have a sense of belonging in their local community.

For author Tim Winton, the sea has transformed him into a steward helping to save one of the last wild places in the world, Ningaloo Reef.

Writing this book changed me too. Spending time with Indigenous academic Dr Chels Marshall and the Erub artists of the Torres Strait helped me see the world in a different light; they gave me a precious glimpse of just how visceral their connection to sea country is.

The power of the ocean is brought home to me every afternoon these days, as I watch a surfer's calm settle over my teenage son after he's been out in the big sets, getting his daily fix of 'the great poultice', as Tim Winton calls it.

The boundless sea around us, it seems, has a gift for everyone.

I hope you find these stories as unforgettable as I do.

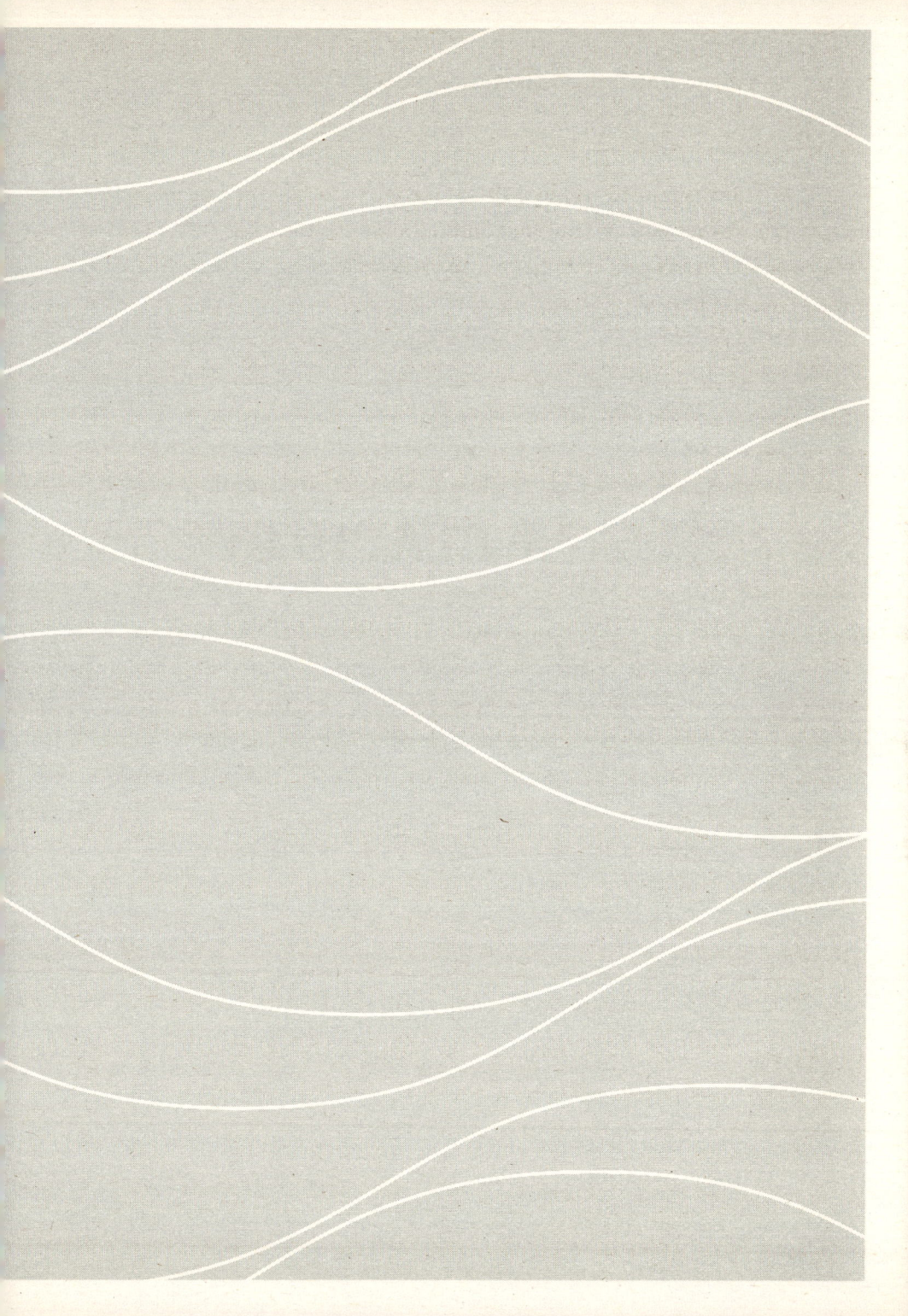

CHAPTER 1

LAYNE BEACHLEY

High Tide

~~~

THE ROAR OF the Pacific breakers greets you as you walk into the Northern Beaches home of seven-time world surfing champion Layne Beachley. Her husband, INXS star Kirk Pengilly, is watching Sunday afternoon rugby league in the living room, and in the garage on a giant board rack is her quiver of 40 surfboards that she stores at home (she has 102 in total at last count). They are objects of beauty – sleek, curved, shell coloured. Her current favourite is particularly beautiful: an MG, shaped for her by the legendary Mauricio Gil, whose shop in nearby Brookvale is crammed with boards named the Zipper, Magic Carpet or the Slayer. 'It has a blue resin pattern on it,' Layne says. 'I really love it, I've found my groove on it.'

She walks up a set of stairs leading to her office: a spacious eyrie with an expansive view over Freshwater Beach. During lockdown, with time on her hands, Layne started building a self-empowerment platform called Awake Academy, an online course based on some of the life lessons she's learned as a professional athlete. One look at the multicoloured Post-it Notes on the walls, and the spiritual classics on her bookshelf – Eckhart Tolle's *The Power of Now* and Neale Donald Walsch's *Conversations with God* – and it's obvious that she is pouring her usual zeal into her new business.

Her sunny, confident nature works well when she is on stage presenting, and she enjoys it. The course itself, she is keen to point out, is not simply about reaching your potential; there's a strong emphasis on self-awareness and self-care. 'One of my favourite topics is incorporating what I call the seven doctors into your day: drinking lots of water, exercise, healthy food, sunshine, rest, laughter and journalling.'

If anyone has learned the importance of self-care, it's Layne. She's painfully aware of how hard she's driven herself and the havoc it's wrought on her body and mind as she battled her way to the top of a tough, male-dominated sport. She has regular chiropractic sessions for her neck, back and hips, injuries caused from pushing her body too hard, and has spent so many hours out in the ocean straddling a surfboard

~~~

She has spent so many hours out in the ocean straddling a surfboard that it has changed her physiology.

~~~

that it has changed her physiology; she finds it almost impossible to stand with her legs together, and her upper body has a slight curve from countless hours of paddling.

'I placed ferociously unrealistic expectations on myself for a long time,' she says. 'For many years I rarely took care of myself and I was only focused on my goals and achievements. I have a very high tolerance for discomfort, but for many years it was at the expense of being a well-rounded human being. I neglected my body signals and pushed through the pain.' She pours cups of herbal tea: she might be a tough competitor but she is a warm and hospitable host.

'I had no empathy and no compassion for myself, which stems from my upbringing as well. My dad's been a wonderful inspiration – he was an incredibly fit man – and I just adored him, and still do, but the tough love approach he took to parenting ended up having a long-lasting impact.'

When she reflects on the lengths to which she pushed her body on the surfing circuit, she grows serious. 'I acquired a tiger shark mentality. I saw the breaking down of my mind and body as just another challenge that I had to push through and overcome. The more broken I became, the harder I worked. I would just keep pushing myself until I ended up depressed and scared and very isolated.'

As well as suffering from chronic fatigue syndrome, she endured some very dark days of clinical depression, which led, at one particularly low moment, to the brink of suicide. A herniated disc in her neck in 2005, when she was 33, was the final wake-up call, forcing her to stop surfing for several months and take stock of her life. Since then, Layne has adopted a much more balanced approach, surfing for the sheer pleasure of it, rather than to win.

So what drove her to such extreme measures to prove herself? Layne pauses for a long while before answering; she's thought about this a great deal. When Layne was seven years old, a skinny tomboy with a mop of long blonde hair who was never far from a skateboard, a bike or a surfboard, her mother, Valerie, died of a brain haemorrhage. It was sudden, after a minor operation went wrong.

Soon afterwards, her father, Neil – worried that others would break the news to her – decided to tell her she was adopted. Layne didn't say anything at the time, but the news had a profound impact on her. 'When Dad told me I was adopted, I decided I was going to be the best in the world at something,' she wrote in her journal. 'I just had to be the best to be loved and approved of.'

The mystery of her birth mother and why she had given her up – and the loss of her adoptive mother on top of that – cast a shadow over many of her formative years. The best way, she felt, to deal with such a gaping hole – the search for her true identity, and her need for love and approval – was to channel all her energy and passion into surfing.

It was her great good fortune, she says, to be adopted into a beach-loving family. One of her first memories as a toddler was standing on her brother's skateboard while their father towed her along the beachfront with a towel. She was four years old when she started surfing – Nippers, the surf education classes held every Sunday morning, held no interest for her. Instead, she paddled out the back of the sets at Manly Beach on her foam surfboard. Neil, a keen surfer and member of the local Surf Life Saving club, would be either with her or watching from the club's balcony with a sausage sandwich and a beer.

'As far as I was concerned the lifeguards were the enemy because they just put the flags up where the best waves were,' she recalls. (Surfers are not allowed between the flags.) 'I rode a foamy for nine years. Even then I was so goal oriented. I just remember setting a goal to be on a fibreglass board by sixteen.'

Her competitive streak saw her leave the security of her 'foamie' and the south end – or family end – of the beach and strike out among the boys at the north end. She was the only girl out there. They gave her a hard time, and she was harassed a lot, but she was quick-witted and held her own. Surfing with the best male surfers would sharpen her skills, she knew, so she was always prepared to take a deep breath and surf in their territory. She slowly began making her way up the pecking order for the best waves.

Taking on the boys at the north end was tough, but it still didn't prepare her for the rampant chauvinism involved in representing her school in Year Ten in the national schools title. They gave her such a hard time on the trip to Bells Beach, in Victoria, that it turned her off amateur surfing for life. 'The guys gave me so much trouble, they really hurt me deeply,' she writes in her autobiography, *Beneath the Waves*. One guy even left a condom on her hotel pillow, with a note saying, *I'm in room so and so, see you later*.

Once she'd finished high school, she joined the long hard slog of the professional women's circuit. Unlike the men, the female competitors had no one to pick them up from the airport or station, and there was certainly no fancy accommodation. They stayed in backpacker hostels, and made their own way to their competitions, on planes, trains and buses, often in countries where they didn't speak the language. A surfing coach or lucrative sponsor was something they could only dream about.

Even when she was ranked number two in the world, Layne held down four jobs, working 60-hour weeks to fund her surfing. It was gruelling. And it was incredibly galling, to be treated like a second-class citizen. 'There was an incredible lack of respect for women,' she says. 'We were treated so dismally. We had to surf in poor waves while the best conditions were reserved for the men.'

Layne was one of several trailblazers, alongside Wendy Botha, Pam Burridge and Pauline Menczer, who harnessed their anger about their treatment to advocate for a better deal for women's surfing. Astoundingly, it wasn't until 2018 that female surfers received equal pay. And it was prompted by a photo, which went viral. It showed the two winners of a junior championship holding cheques – the boy's winnings double the amount of the girl's.

Despite all these obstacles, Layne's addiction to surfing has never wavered. On a family holiday with her father and brother, she saw Hawaii's big breaks for the first time – the fabled Sunset Beach, Pipeline and Waimea Bay. They seized her imagination. 'Sunset always had this magical allure for me: it was so threatening, but so beautiful. From the moment I sat down and looked at it, I couldn't take my eyes off it,' she says.

When she was forging her way to the top of women's surfing, she fell in love with Ken Bradshaw, the Hawaiian big wave rider. He greatly admired how she would get out there and tackle the monster swells – swells so big that some of the girls would throw up on the beach because they were so afraid paddling out into them. 'Sunset is one of those places that will kick your arse more than most other places,' Layne says, laughing, 'but will also give you the biggest adrenaline thrill of your life.'

Ken taught her how to read swell charts and how waves are generated. He taught her how to put herself under extreme pressure and enjoy it. 'He taught me to get comfortable with being completely slaughtered, and how to mitigate distraction.' Ken also passed on his passion for tow-in surfing, which introduced her to the outer reefs of Hawaii and the biggest waves of her life. Once, she caught a 15-metre wave – the biggest wave a woman had ever caught at that time – and she was euphoric for days. 'I was in the zone,' she says. 'I'm a Gemini so I always have a million thoughts, but on that wave, my internal dialogue was silenced.'

She'll never forget that ride. As she says in her memoir:

From the speed I was travelling just to catch the wave, I was going at probably forty to fifty kilometres per hour on my feet and I knew it was the biggest wave I'd ever ridden in my life. When I let go of the rope and slowed down to the speed of the wave and the wave caught up to me, because you've got to go faster to catch it, it was like time stood still. My presence of mind had never been so clear. Because I was that scared, my awareness was so in the moment that there was nothing going on. Time stood still and you could hear everything, but you couldn't hear anything. It was a deafening silence. It was one of the most phenomenal experiences where I felt so instantly present.

So what does she do when she gets scared out there in a big swell? 'I acknowledge that I'm scared – as opposed to thinking, Harden the fuck up. I look for an exit strategy such as catching a wave, paddling around to the next beach or getting caught in the impact zone to wash me in. Then I will distract myself by singing the first song that comes to mind, or laugh, or I might share my fear with other surfers. If there is someone out in the water that I get a chance to talk

~~~

'I know I'm equipped, I'm
confident to find my way
out of a situation like that,
but it's also about accepting
my fate and the fact that
the ocean is far more
powerful than me. You have
to constantly respect it,
pay attention to it.'

~~~

to, I'll say, "Hey can you just keep an eye on me?" Often, they're probably scared too.' Sometimes she chants a mantra, like 'I am strong, I am competent, I am experienced, I am knowledgeable. I am equipped to deal with this.'

She's come close to drowning a couple of times. Once, when she was in Fiji, she got wiped out and was held down by the turbulence of a big wave for about 40 seconds. Her girlfriends paddled over, ready to pull her out. 'I remember getting thrashed around under water, unable to fight against it or make my way to the surface. My board was still attached to my ankle, tombstoning on the surface, while I was stuck on the bottom of the ocean.' ('Tombstoning' is when the board is pulled under water by the tail but the nose is up in the air, swaying side to side.) 'It was only 40 seconds, but from down below, it felt like a long time under there. Fortunately, I didn't panic.'

What did that teach her? 'I know I'm equipped, I'm confident to find my way out of a situation like that, but it's also about accepting my fate and the fact that the ocean is far more powerful than me. You have to constantly respect it, pay attention to it. These moments make me realise that life is very fragile.'

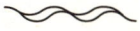

As she perfected her technique and surfed the biggest waves in the world, her longing to meet her biological mother continued to grow. When she was in her early twenties a family friend had taken her to the Births Deaths and Marriages Registry to collect the paperwork to find her birth mother. Layne kept putting off lodging it, though, unsure if she wanted to open her heart to someone she had never known.

When Layne finally met her, it was with a mixture of complex emotions. Maggie Gardner had been trying to find her daughter for years, and finally got in touch when Layne was 27 years old, after she had won her first world championship and was months away from claiming her second one.

Layne's first feeling was relief, when she found out why her mother had given her up. Maggie had been only sixteen, an unwed girl from a strict family, when she realised she was pregnant. She was forced by her father to give up her baby for adoption. But when Layne discovered the circumstances of her conception, she was deeply shocked. Maggie had been raped after a dinner date with the manager of a Kings Cross modelling agency.

After a tumultuous start to their relationship – Maggie admitted her unintentionally clumsy approach was a textbook case of how *not* to go about reaching one's daughter – the pair became very fond of each other and Maggie became a fixture in Layne's life. Maggie passed away from ovarian cancer in 2017. Her other daughter, Melissa, is now close with Layne.

There are many famous surfers who have had a positive impact on Layne's life – Tom Carroll, Wendy Botha, Barton Lynch and Pam Burridge all spring quickly to mind. But it is the ocean that has had the most powerful effect. The big blue has always been her comfort, her consolation, her retreat and her escape from the world. It's where she recharges and where she celebrates her wins.

Right from the start, Layne was aware of the solace of salt water. As she writes in her teenage journal:

If I had my surfboard that's all that I needed – and my bikini. It gave me an escape from all troubles. It was such a safe environment. There were times when I went out and I solved all my problems. And I'd feel reconnected, because I'd processed frustration or whatever was going on in my system. And then there were times where I'd go out there to escape it and think about it and not worry – not try to solve my problems. That's the wonder of it.

It's the place that nurtures me, reflects me, teaches me a lot. It's like going to Mother Nature. It's where I feel the safest. It's the only place I feel safe enough. No one is around to see me cry or laugh or scream or yell. If you scream under water no one can hear you.

Today, she remains just as convinced of its transformative qualities. A storm is brewing out to sea and she's keeping a close eye on it, wondering if she'll get a chance to sneak in a quick surf before nightfall. You can almost feel her quivering with anticipation.

'The biggest lesson I've learned from the ocean is surrender. Because I'm a control freak. The ocean is a great place for control freaks. I've learned to surrender to a force more powerful than me. I've learned respect and admiration, and how it reflects my emotions. If I paddle out feeling cocky and arrogant, it will slap me across the face. It will just frustrate me, as if to say, "wake up!"

'But then, on the other hand, when I'm paddling towards a wave and I think this is going to kick my arse and it doesn't, it tells me: you need to lighten up today. I could be projecting but that is the process I go through mentally when I'm in the water. I'm often out there when it's big. I'm often out there on my own. It's a great reflection point on channelling my own fears, addressing them, and overcoming them.'

Spending most of her life out in the ocean has afforded Layne many interactions with its creatures. She has had the privilege of swimming with whale sharks in Western Australia. She's been within 3 metres of a humpback whale. She's swum among hammerhead sharks in the Galapagos Islands, and with turtles in Tahiti, and with more dolphins than she can remember. Each time she pinches herself at her good fortune.

~~~

**'The biggest lesson
I've learned from the
ocean is surrender.'**

~~~

'Dolphins are incredibly playful, they dropped in on me on a wave once, and another time they pretended they were sharks, hurtling towards me, then they jumped up on either side of me as if to say, surprise! They're very playful, very mischievous – and fabulous surfers, of course.'

Her most extraordinary close encounter with marine life, perhaps, was when an orca joined her and a group of other surfers in Hawaii, when they were lined up out the back, waiting for the waves to come. Orcas are formidable creatures: on average 7 metres long and weighing 4000 kilograms. They are renowned for being killing machines when they hunt in packs. 'We were in this particular spot right in front of my house that Ken and I shared at Sunset Beach, and this orca swam in and started slapping its tail on the surface of the water. It was so loud that Ken could hear it, and feel the vibrations, from the house 100 metres away. It was as if the ocean honoured its presence. Everything went flat and quiet.'

When it comes to sharks, Layne respects that she is surfing in their domain. 'It's their territory, their playground, their home,' she says. She'll often stay out in the water when the shark alarm goes off, because the risk of being attacked is incredibly slim. 'Sharks aren't out to get us; they're just going about their business. It's almost always a case of mistaken identity if there is an attack – the person has accidentally swum near a food source or a bait ball [a dense group of fish] and the shark has mistaken them for a seal or a large fish.'

She's passionate about the eradication of shark nets. 'All they do is catch and kill other marine life for the sharks to pick off, like a buffet. It's usually harmless marine life like turtles, dolphins and rays. It's such antiquated technology. Non-lethal measures such as drone surveillance, alert systems, personal shark deterrents and shark-smart devices are much more effective at keeping people safe without the cost to marine life.'

It saddens her greatly to see the damage we are doing to the ocean. 'When I started surfing in the late '70s, the south-east winds used to blow all the pollution around the North Head of Manly. It was disgusting, it smelled like raw sewage. That's cleaned up a lot but the water is unseasonably warm now. We're not getting those cold currents like we used to.

'I've also noticed a tremendous amount of plastic on the beaches, which I'd never seen before. There are more whales, but far less fish and marine life. I have such a heavy heart when I think about this planet. The ocean covers more than 70 per cent of our planet. If it was a person, we would treat it with much more respect.' There are lots of small things we can do to help, she says. On the way back from the beach, she picks up every piece of plastic that she sees, from cigarette butts to plastic bags.

At 52, Layne has found a way to get the balance just right. She surfs on average six days a week – she has the luxury and freedom to surf whenever she feels like it. It takes three minutes to run to Freshwater Beach with one of her boards and five and a half to Queenscliff. If the first 40 years of her aquatic life were about seeking love and approval by being the most successful female surfer in history, and winning at all costs, the last decade has been far more gentle. When she heads out for a surf these days, it's more about experiencing the joy of being in the water, and in the moment, feeling the power of the waves and the solace of the salt.

As she put it in her journal:

It's time I go surfing for the love of it. Remove the mind, the expectations, the pressure, the desire to win. Replace it with all the desire to experience joy, the joy and relaxation of being in the solace of the ocean, enjoying the intoxicating power of the wave, the laughter of my heart and the clarity of my mind.

Her passion for surfing is infectious. She's a director at the new wave pool at Sydney Olympic Park, URBNSURF, and has attracted lots of girls to her local Boardriders club at Freshwater; she offers free coaching sessions if they become members. If there is one thing she'd love to convey to others about the ocean it's 'the way it will hold you. There's no reason to fear it.'

Despite the scars and injuries, surfing has had a potent long-term effect on her psychologically. 'I feel more unconditionally calm and supported,' she says. A happy marriage helps too. 'When we first started going out, we almost needed couples therapy because Kirk didn't really like the sunshine or sand or the water,' she laughs. They're teaching each other a lot. 'He's taught me tenderness, nurturing, love, how to be more empathic, compassionate.' She's taught him, among many other things, how to live a much healthier life.

If she could go back in time and give herself some advice as a young woman, what would it be? She doesn't need any time to consider it. 'Lighten up! Success doesn't have to be hard work and pain, you can enjoy yourself, and have a lot of fun along the way as well.' She picks up the tea mugs and heads downstairs to see Kirk. 'You don't have to take things so seriously.'

CHAPTER 2

JAMES PITTAR

On a Clear Day

～～～

FEW ATHLETES CAN rival marathon swimmer James Pittar when it comes to iron will. Twenty-five years ago, when he was twenty-eight, he joined the elite coterie of swimmers who have managed to carve their way across the ocean for fourteen hours straight without a break, to cross the English Channel.

Twelve hours into his swim, when most people would probably have been close to breaking point, his coach Narelle Simpson asked him to dig deep and find the strength to swim as fast as he could for the next 500 metres. The goal?

To reach a sandbar. If he made it in time, the changing tide on the other side would propel him towards the French shore in two hours rather than six. James put his head down, swam like a demon, and made it.

He staggered out of the water a few hours later, covered in Vaseline against the cold, his legs shaking with exhaustion. After his feat had been certified by an official observer, he fell into the arms of Narelle and his mother.

What makes his accomplishment even more astonishing is the fact that James is almost completely blind. 'He can't see a thing out there,' Narelle says. 'I don't think I've ever met anyone who has the same dogged determination and tenacity that James has. He just never gives up.'

James began losing his sight when he was fifteen, when he was in Year Eight. He had retinitis pigmentosa, a rare, degenerative disease that gradually destroys the retina at the back of the eye. By the time he was 25 he had almost no vision.

To say it's distressing to slowly lose your sight as a teenager, when you are finding your way in the world and yearning for independence, would be a huge understatement. 'It was hard not to be frightened,' James recalls. 'I wanted to do all the usual things most young men wanted to do at that stage. I wanted to go to the pub, get a job, go to university, hopefully meet a nice girl. How was I going to do all that if I couldn't see?'

James sits in the back studio of his Northern Beaches home. He is a warm and erudite host, and is candid about the

'I wanted to go to the pub, get a job, go to university, hopefully meet a nice girl. How was I going to do all that if I couldn't see?'

challenges of being blind. 'Where was I going to live? How would my friends handle me being blind? Would I have to carry a cane? What was my life going to be like if I couldn't read? And couldn't play sport?'

Sport had always been important in the Pittar family: his grandmother had represented England in hockey, and as a boy James had played rugby, cricket and tennis, and surfed most weekends at Freshwater Beach on Sydney's North Shore with his father and older brother Tony.

In the 1980s, schools and universities were less inclusive than they are today, and as James's sight deteriorated, his parents began to consider withdrawing him from Shore School, the Church of England Grammar School he had been attending. Should their son be going to a school for the blind instead? A meeting with the headmaster of the school at the time, the late Basil Travers, set them straight.

'Does James enjoy coming here?' Travers asked the couple.

'Yes, he loves it,' they told him.

'Well, God didn't make everyone equal,' Travers said. 'If he wants to stay at this school then he can. We'll make it work.'

Then, in a move that was revolutionary at the time, the school installed a reading machine provided by James's father. It displayed a large-print version of his school books on a TV monitor. The school also ensured James was not disadvantaged in his assessments: during exam time, a Year Eleven boy would read out the questions for him in his own separate room. By adapting to new technology, and giving James the chance to participate, Shore helped him to continue at school and hold his own with the other students.

James credits those years at Shore as instilling in him a sense of resilience and discipline that he has drawn on all his life. 'Instead of being in a blind school, I was expected to compete with 160 other able-bodied students,' he says. 'It was tough, but it gave me the inner strength to face a lot of obstacles in life.' It helped, too, that his family was hugely supportive. Ironically, his father was an ophthalmologist and his mother an orthoptist, before her two sons were born.

But as James's world grew darker, and smaller, he began missing sport acutely. He needed it more than ever to feel connected with others. His dream to represent Australia in cricket or football was already shattered. A blind game of soccer, as he put it, 'is a pretty violent affair'. He enjoyed rowing, and did well at it. But it was when he began flexing his swimming muscles, churning up and down the lanes of the pool, that he began to shine. Within a few months of competitive swimming he was representing Australia in the disabled swimming championships. When he took to the ocean, and began swimming in vast tracts of salt water, life suddenly blossomed. In the ocean, he could compete with able-bodied people. Ocean swimming opened up the world for him – quite literally.

'He may not be able to see the marine life or coral or seaweed,' Narelle says, 'but out in the ocean, he is free. He can be in control. There is nothing to bump into – no gutters, no doors, no poles in the street. Out here he can move around, as fast as he wants, and feel at ease. It gives him incredible peace of mind.'

It was Narelle who first suggested he swim the English Channel. A lot of people scoffed at the idea, but she knew he had it in him. After several years of working together, Narelle had instilled enough self-belief in James for him to rise to the challenge.

The year-long preparations were daunting: gruelling weekly long-distance swims at large Olympic pools, and a four- to five-hour ocean or lake swim every weekend. He trained every day at his parents' small backyard swimming pool as well, by tethering himself to a fence post, for up to three hours at time. He churned through the water right through winter, even in the rain, whatever the conditions and regardless of how he was feeling. Then there was all the paperwork needed to persuade the Channel Swimming Association to allow a blind person to enter the race. All the effort was worth it. 'Crossing the English Channel was monumental,' Narelle says, 'in the sense that it allowed him to start seeing the world – via the oceans.'

One of his first conquests after the English Channel was the elite, and even more daunting, Manhattan Island Marathon Swim – a 46-kilometre race around Manhattan Island that navigates boats, strong tides and pollution. Not to mention corpses, body parts, animal remains and large logs that are often found in the waters. The New York City race took so much out of him both physically and psychologically that he was almost in tears as he clambered up the ladder at the finish, looking over his shoulder to the Statue of Liberty.

Then he swam from Perth to Rottnest Island in a swell so big it made him seasick. Only 300 of 2000 competitors finished the race that day. Next, he tackled the Bering Strait, between northern Russia and Alaska – without a wetsuit, in water that was 5 degrees Celsius. The oceans encircling the US followed. While most tourists prepare for travel with a list of places to visit, James had just one goal in each country: to swim its oceans, as fast as humanly possible.

The most challenging marathon James ever swam was close to home, across the Cook Strait between the North and South islands of New Zealand. There, the swells were so enormous, and the temperature dropped so fast, that his team almost forfeited the race.

'People said it was good that I didn't see what was happening that day because I probably would have given it away,' he says, shifting his legs and tapping his hand on the table in front of him. In their inflatable boat, his team put their life jackets on and fought hard to keep circling around him. They were catapulted up and over 4-metre waves, buffeted by a fierce 65-kilometre per hour wind, and kept losing sight of him.

About 500 metres from the rocks of the North Island, the race helicopter started monitoring the group. The seas were so mountainous they discussed declaring the swim over and winching James to safety. But one of his support crew, former US water polo player and marathon swimmer Chad Schneider, dived overboard and, putting his body on the line, went to help him reach the shore. He put his arms around James just as a massive wave scooped them up and sent them crashing onto the rocks. 'There are the rocks, mate,' Chad told him. 'You've made it.' The pair then turned around and swam another 100 metres towards the crew, who picked them up and threw them, both shaking, onto the floor of the boat. The two have since become firm friends.

So does he get scared out in the deep, especially as he can't see? 'No,' he says. 'My job is the easiest of everyone's – all I have to do is swim. It's my team that carries the burden of motivating me, feeding me, making sure I'm heading in the right direction, making sure I am safe, all the while paddling, using a megaphone and battling seasickness. They've got all the responsibility. They've got my life in their hands.'

From their inflatable boat, or from Narelle's kayak, they watch over him like a hawk. Directions are given by a whistle: one blast for left, and two short ones for right. ('And three long blasts for a shark,' as James likes to include in his speeches for a laugh.) In the English Channel, his team use a megaphone. The Channel swim does not allow a swimmer to touch anyone in the boat, so they use a long pole to feed him with an open-ended syringe for his carbohydrate fuel, and a water bottle.

Every year without fail, whatever the weather, James and Chad swim the Coogee Island Challenge, out around Wedding Cake Island and back. The pair were in a convivial mood recently as they joined the queue of hundreds waiting to race. James explains that he swims with Chad to his right. If James bumps into him, he veers to the left. If he needs to veer right, Chad will tap him on his right leg. He will hold both ankles if he needs James to stop. Sometimes, he says, there are advantages to being blind. 'I've never worried about sharks because I can't see them.'

Most importantly, his team are there to prop him up psychologically when he's about to throw in the towel. 'They know that after eight hours, it is almost inevitable that I'll start to lose it. I start swimming erratically, just heading in the wrong direction. I can't understand their directions even if they're using a megaphone. I just lose the plot.' They know if they keep encouraging him he will come good.

Much of marathon swimming is a mental game, he says. 'Keeping distracted, not letting boredom get the better of you, is half the battle.' Sometimes this involves his team reading supportive emails from home from their boat.

Swimming around six continents, and growing more confident in himself and his abilities each year, gave James the self-belief to start dating. He was 34 when he met Jenny, after being urged to go online by his friend. His eyes light up when he describes meeting 'the love of his life'. 'I'll

~~~

'My job is the easiest of
everyone's – all I have to do
is swim. It's my team that
carries the burden ... They've
got my life in their hands.'

~~~

always remember the night I found her,' he writes in his autobiography, *Blind Vision*. 'She was into scuba diving and travelling, and I could sense a kindness in her profile. I had to know more!'

They hit it off straight away.

'She was so relaxed and easygoing and wasn't bothered by the fact that I was blind. We just had so much to talk about – it felt like we'd known each other for a long time – and the physical attraction was strong,' he writes. Six months later they were married and moving in together. 'It seems a strange concept to me now that I'd ever lived without her.'

As much as he sings the praises of his family and team, James can only achieve what he does through true grit. Narelle, who has trained swimmers of Olympic calibre, considers James 'one of the elites'. 'He's one of a group of very special swimmers who has the right stuff. He also just happens to be blind,' she says. 'He's always had the most incredibly gutsy attitude. His motto is not to win but to finish the race. He's a plodder, but he's unbelievably tenacious. Once he's set his mind to doing something he just does not give in. The outcome is not as important to him as getting out there, over and over again, and pushing himself to the very limits of his ability. He has a slightly obsessive-compulsive tendency and a hyper focus that all marathon swimmers need. He swims with his heart and his mind as much as physical stamina.'

'James is the epitome of success,' Chad says, his cap pulled down firmly against the glare of a hot summer's day in Coogee. 'He does not let his disability impact his desire to achieve.' The pair share a similar outlook: it is not winning the race that counts, but whether you push yourself to do your absolute best. They met in 2003, while competing in the Rottnest Channel Swim, a notoriously difficult stretch of water in Western Australia. After bashing his way through 3-metre swells, James was disqualified on a technicality. Chad was flabbergasted. 'He was the first blind swimmer to finish, he was absolutely elated, and he'd turned up year after year. I just couldn't believe their decision. I said to James, "It doesn't matter if they don't write your name up in the paper and you didn't go home with an embroidered shirt. You know that you made it."'

As well as admiring James's stoicism, Chad simply loves swimming with him. 'We have a great synergy when we swim together, and we have a lot of fun. I like getting my James fix.' Both are sports mad and love going to the cricket together, and James is now the ambassador for Chad's swimming school. The Coogee Island Challenge is usually followed by their annual 'burger bet' at the Coogee Bay Hotel. This year the New York Yankees defeated James's favourite team, the Boston Red Sox, so Chad collected his burger winnings.

'Something wonderful usually happens when you hang out with James,' he says. One day, as James's guide, he found himself swimming alongside Australian swimming great Murray Rose. Another day, when they were at the cricket, ABC Radio asked James to call the match. 'So James starts commentating live, and it's unbelievably accurate. His other senses, such as his hearing, have become magnified since he lost his sight. He could tell by listening to which side of the cricket ground the crowd was cheering the loudest, and the sound of the bat as to where the ball was going. He's a remarkable person.'

Those who work with James tend to stay with him. Narelle began coaching him in 1993 and finds it a helpful reminder of what we are all capable of. She realised she had a particular flair for teaching people with disabilities early in her career as a coach. 'Everyone looks at what they can't do, but I tend to look at what they can do instead.' You learn so much, she says, particularly how to be flexible. The narrow-mindedness of other swimmers astounds her.

'There are people who don't know what to do when a blind person swims over them accidentally in the pool. I say to them, "Could you just stop and think about it a bit more? Could you wait for him to be at the other end, then start? Could you swim around him? Why can't you be a little more patient?" I often say to the ones who are the most intolerant: "Why don't you try and swim with your eyes closed?" I wish everyone could attempt swimming with goggles blackened out. It might give them a better sense of what it feels like to be blind.'

She loves that blind swimmers like James use their other senses, such as being highly attuned to the currents, the tides and the weather. They count their strokes in the pool. They feel the water around them, and work out how close they are to the wall by the feel of the backwash. There is always a way to deal with a situation, though it may not be immediately obvious, she says.

James always finds a way to navigate. He can tell from the coolness of the water where he is – for instance, it will get warmer when he approaches Shelly Beach, near Manly. The wind and the currents – even the strongest – can also be used to his advantage. 'I love bashing against the waves. I love the thrill of it when it's choppy, that you're going to get absolutely whacked out there, and that you might be smacked in the face. I like using the wind as a directional tool. If I can feel the wind blowing over my head, I know that when I turn around and come back I am going to have the wind behind me and it's going to be a fast trip home.'

The ocean remains one of the great mainstays in James's life. 'I love how unpredictable it is, from the most benign conditions to the most treacherous. It can be placid as a lake one day, but then 7-foot swells the next. It can be a painful battle against the current, against the wind, and against the cross swell.'

His feet always walk towards the sea in times of trouble. When his hero and supporter, the great English Channel

~~~

Blind swimmers like James use their other senses, such as being highly attuned to the currents, the tides and the weather.

~~~

swimmer Des Renford, died of a heart attack at 72, he sought refuge in the salt water. Likewise when his great mate Ched Towns died of altitude sickness trying to climb Mount Everest. Swimming in the ocean, as he writes in his book, 'released all the misery and helplessness' he'd been feeling. He would emerge from the water 'renewed, and happy for the first time in weeks'.

These days, James is more interested in swimming to benefit others than in winning medals or smashing records. The Fred Hollows Foundation, set up to continue the work of the late, great Australian professor of ophthalmology, which has helped restore the sight of millions around the world, is a cause that is close to his heart. Each year James raises money and awareness about the foundation by walking or swimming; one of his early fundraising swims in 2011, Malabar Beach to Bondi, was for the cause. 'I love knowing that by swimming I'm helping people on the other side of the world to see – whether they are in Nepal, Pakistan, Eritrea or Ethiopia. It's very gratifying.'

What he especially loves is the tangible effects of their work. It is $25 to restore someone's sight. And this helps more than one person. In the developing world, it's often girls and young women who are carers of the visually impaired; restoring someone's sight frees up their family to continue at school or university or to go back to work.

James is passionate about improving the sight – and health – of First Nations People. He was shocked when he discovered that trachoma and cataracts are rampant in many First Peoples' communities. 'I couldn't believe we are some of the most affluent countries in the world and we can't even provide basic health care to Traditional Owners of the land.'

He also adores helping out with the Rainbow Club, which teaches water skills and safety to youngsters with disabilities and special needs. 'Learning to swim in Australia is not a privilege, it's a right. Everyone deserves a fair go, especially when it comes to enjoying all our beautiful beaches and oceans.'

Spending so much time in the sea has given him a keen sense of the devastating results of climate change. When he swam in Phuket, Thailand, eighteen months after the 2004 tsunami, the community was just beginning to rebuild. Only 120 metres from the sand was a six-lane road with buildings on the other side. The road was still closed due to damage. 'You could imagine what it would have done. There were power lines not far away.'

What would he most like to see if his sight could be somehow restored? He answers without hesitation: the faces of his wife and his daughter. He beams with pride when he talks about his daughter, and how she's become interested in ocean swimming. He hopes he can pass on to her the enormous respect he has for the ocean.

'The ocean is not forgiving at all. If you take it for granted, it will come back to bite you hard. It has such an incredible power to it, it can be lethal. We've seen what can happen in yachting races like the Sydney to Hobart, in those monumental wind and waves.' The disastrous 1998 race resulted in the death of six sailors, the sinking of five yachts and 55 participants being rescued by helicopter. 'Spending so much time in the water has made me humble. No matter how much you study it, no matter how fit you are, or how well you plan a trip, you simply cannot control it. It's wild and unpredictable. I never underestimate its powers.'

During a swim from Shelly Beach to Collaroy Beach, the conditions were so bad that James and his coach Matthew Logan, who was kayaking alongside him, almost had to turn around. All Matthew could see was 200 metres of white water. It was getting dark. It began to rain. They were bracing themselves for a gruelling six-hour swim back when a fisherman picked them up and took them back to shore. 'Things can turn nasty very quickly.'

Although he doesn't see himself as a spiritual person, being in the water for so many years has fine-tuned his appreciation of nature and the complex, if sometimes unseen, way we are all connected. He was always very close to his grandmother, who was an outstanding sportswoman. He admired her unwaveringly positive attitude to life; she, in turn, was an avid fan of his swimming feats.

Several times, during his most arduous marathons, when his spirits have begun to flag, and he's felt psychologically beaten, he's noticed a seagull hovering closely overhead.

'When a gull hovers over me like that when I'm out in the middle of the ocean, I feel like that's her spirit saying "Well done, James. You've done me proud."'

CHAPTER 3

VALERIE TAYLOR

Playing
with Sharks

~~~

VALERIE TAYLOR, THE underwater filmmaker who, along with her late husband, Ron, probably helped change our perception of sharks more than anyone else, has just returned home to Sydney from her final dive trip. It was, fittingly, in one of the most stunning places to dive on the planet: Raja Ampat, Indonesia, in a body of water studded with high islands and brilliantly hued corals. As she dived within this underwater empire, she reached out to stroke the morays, as other people might stroke their pet dog or cat.

'Some fish like a gentle touch,' she says. 'They like to be tickled if you're gentle enough. Marine animals don't want to harm you. They only wish to defend themselves. So if you're very gentle and talk to them, they let you interact with them.'

Valerie's diving days might now be over but she will continue to snorkel – 'preferably near the equator, in water about 29 degrees'. She'll go with her nephew, Mark, who operates a dive vessel in the warm Indonesian waters. One of the many benefits of being immersed in salt water is that it makes her feel young again. 'Above water I feel like an old lady, but underwater, I feel like I'm about 40,' she says. 'Gravity drags me down on land but once I'm in the water I feel I can fly anywhere. I can see something and just fly over, like a bird, towards it.'

Life in and around the ocean has left her with physical scars. She's been bitten four times by sharks: once dangerously, when she was filming off San Diego. There, the Coast Guard helicopter winched her to safety and flew her to hospital, where a plastic surgeon stitched the gashed leg together. It was a useful lesson: if you get bitten by a shark, Valerie tells fellow divers, make sure you are working for Hollywood. Her skin has been 'ruined from sitting in a tinny in the sun for way too long' during her youth. And one of her eardrums is damaged, from a charter that went wrong when a bunch of drunken footballers thought it would be amusing to pull everyone from their bunks and throw them in the water.

Still, though Valerie would deny it, decades of being in salt water have imbued her with a life-bright presence; she almost seems to glow like the phosphorescence she's dived among. Spending so long in the aquatic world has also left her with a fierce determination to protect its creatures.

Her apartment in Fairlight has glorious views out over Sydney Harbour towards the South Head. Here, she often hosts other activists, such as volunteers from the Australian Marine Conservation Society. They're as determined as Valerie to get rid of the shark nets that have been put up along many of the beaches on the eastern coast of Australia.

'If I achieve one thing before I die, it will be to see an end to the shark nets,' she says. 'They're evil. The marine life that gets caught in them is just appalling. Ron and I have rescued turtles, dugongs, manta rays, gropers and whales from the nets up and down the eastern seaboard.' One of the saddest things they ever saw was a baby dolphin that had drowned in one. It had scratches all over it from its mother trying to free it. To her right, as she speaks, is a pair of binoculars that she uses to gaze at the ships. In front of her is a large photo of Ron, who passed away thirteen years ago. She looks at this photo frequently.

Both Valerie and Ron were spearfishers who became dedicated conservationists when they realised the fish they were killing had personalities. Some were timid; others were bold. Some recognised them from previous dives. Their tipping point came one day when they emerged from a spearfishing competition to find the beach covered with beautiful sea creatures 'killed for no good reason', she says, 'other than the thrill of points in a competition'. They resolved that, from this point on, the only thing they would use to shoot a marine animal was a camera.

And with that camera, they became the dynamic duo who documented the underwater world around Australia and brought it into our living rooms. Ron was the technical genius, devising the earliest underwater camera housings. With her blonde ponytail, pink wetsuit and unique ability to understand and befriend marine life, Valerie proved the perfect presenter.

They began by selling mesmerising five-minute clips to television stations. Their fame grew as the footage moved to colour, and became more dramatic and daring. The couple hit the big time soon afterwards, in the early 1970s, when Hollywood came calling. Out of the blue, Universal Pictures sent them the galley proofs of a manuscript by a debut novelist, Peter Benchley, about a giant rogue shark creating fear and loathing in a resort town on the east coast of the US. The producers wanted to know if Valerie and Ron thought it could be adapted into a movie. Poring over the proofs, the couple saw plenty of work for themselves, and said yes. When Benchley's novel – *Jaws* – went on to become a bestseller, Universal snapped up the rights, and employed a young director called Steven Spielberg to film it.

Spielberg didn't hesitate in asking Valerie and Ron to capture footage of great white sharks. They filmed off Port

~~~

**'Above water I feel like an
old lady, but underwater,
I feel like I'm about 40.'**

~~~

Lincoln, in South Australia, and their dramatic underwater scenes were used in the film. 'We had absolutely no idea how big *Jaws* would be.' She shakes her head, watching a ferry cross the harbour to the North Head. 'And if we'd known the damage it would do to the way people perceived sharks, we probably wouldn't have done it at all.'

Peter Benchley felt much the same. He, Valerie and Ron were horrified at the way the film demonised sharks and prompted countless shark-hunting trips around the world. 'The philosophy for a long time was that the only good shark was a dead shark,' Valerie recalls. 'It was seen as a great sign of masculinity to be holding up a totally harmless 2-metre grey nurse shark off the back of a fishing boat, professing they were saving swimmers from being eaten alive.'

The truth, she says, is that the grey nurse shark would have to be one of the most misunderstood creatures on the planet. There has never been a proven attack on a human by a grey nurse. They are fish eaters. Yet, due to the media's desire for drama, it has wrongly been portrayed as a danger to swimmers.

Both Valerie and Ron knew sharks so well by this stage that they could capture their compelling nature on camera without fear. They knew that if they respected the fact they were in the sharks' domain, and approached them with care, the risk of injury was minimal. On one dive, Valerie even hitched a ride on a grey nurse shark, hanging on to her dorsal fin to cajole her away from their filming area when Ron was shooting with the American Navy. 'Her slow swimming was faster than my fast swimming,' she says matter-of-factly. 'She didn't care.'

Once, Ron resuscitated a shark with his scuba tank as it lay ensnared in a fishing net. 'Ron gave him air from his regulator. We didn't think he was going to make it but he quite suddenly gave a shiver and I could feel his body trying to swim.' It was exhilarating to free them when they were entangled, she says. 'You can feel their great energy, yearning for freedom. They want to be free, just like everyone else. And, like many marine animals, they are far more intelligent than they are often given credit for.' She is sitting on her sofa, browsing through her extraordinary collection of underwater photography. 'I'll never forget the day, off the South Australian coast, when we freed a great white – she swam in a big circle back to Ron, who was in the water, before she swam out to sea. She knew exactly what we'd done. It was her way of saying thanks.' She smiles at the memory, then becomes suddenly animated. 'People didn't understand the importance of the sharks in the marine ecosystem. An abundance of sharks meant an abundance of other marine life.'

After *Jaws* was released – and became a box-office hit – the couple spent several months in the US. They told the public on radio, on television and in print that the shark in *Jaws* was fictional, and that sharks were not out to get us. It was to no avail. 'Sharks were still being seen as evil killing machines, in much the way witches and demons used to be feared.' They began lobbying for the grey nurse shark to be protected. 'Most people supported us when we tried to protect cute marine animals like sea lions and potato cod, but when it came to sharks, it was a different matter.'

Not to be deterred, Valerie set off on a single-minded campaign, writing one letter after another to fisheries and the government, submitting stories to magazines. 'Sharks are just going about their business. They don't come out onto our territory, do they? So if we go into theirs, we should be polite and leave them alone.' It worked. The grey nurse became the first shark in the world to be totally protected by law.

The couple's shark sanctuaries, along with those for giant gropers north of Cairns known as potato cod, are an achievement Valerie's immensely proud of. She was deeply moved when, in 2011, she received an Order of Australia for services to conservation. 'When you love something, you want to care for it,' she told the packed room.

When Ron succumbed to cancer, in 2012, it was the end of life as Valerie knew it. The loss was as grave as if she had lost her arms or legs. 'He was my other half. After so many years of Ron and Valerie Taylor, I now had to learn to be on my own. Just Valerie. For a while there, I didn't know what to do with myself,' she says. The only way forward, and the best way to honour Ron's memory, was to continue the work of their several decades together: conserving life in the ocean.

After a lifetime under the waves, during which she and Ron created several marine sanctuaries where sea creatures can, as she puts it, 'live and love in peace', she is also now working hard to get rid of the shark nets and ensure the protection of grey nurse sharks along the east coast. 'These sharks attract diving tourists from all over the world, and are protected by law, but are still being killed at an alarming rate as bycatch.' By this she is referring to modern fishing methods such as large and strong fishing nets and deep sea trawling, which catch not just the targeted animals but also countless other marine creatures in the process. In order to make a living, the crew of these commercial fishing fleets must turn a blind eye. Perhaps because the intelligence of these marine animals is not truly understood.

Probably more than anyone else in the world, Valerie knows how smart marine life can be. Australian documentary makers Sally Aitken and Bettina Dalton's *Playing with Sharks*, which premiered at the Sundance Film Festival in 2021 and was quickly snapped up by National Geographic, shows fascinating footage of Valerie interacting with her underwater friends. What's striking is how gentle she is, and how the fish respond. Many even show signs of remembering her between visits. For some years, she visited two giant eels, Harry and Fang, off Heron Island. 'I always liked to feed them bits of fish and they would slide around me, begging for more. They love a good but gentle hug.'

Perhaps the closest she has come to actually befriending a sea creature was with sea lions, which, she says, are 'playful, curious and loving'. 'It's such an enormous pleasure diving with

~~~

The only way forward, and the best way to honour Ron's memory, was to continue the work of their several decades together: conserving life in the ocean.

~~~

them,' she writes in her autobiography, *An Adventurous Life*. 'On the surface they waddle about like giant Labrador puppies. Underwater they dart around you, playing quizzical games and playing with each other.'

'They're beautiful creatures,' she says. 'Sometimes they hug you. They come up and put their flippers around you. You've got to watch out because their whiskers are very sharp.' Potato cod, too, she regards as friends. Often they come so close, with their curious faces, that you can reach out and touch them.

And then, of course, there are the whales. While working with the American filmmaker Peter Gimbel, she and Ron lived on a whale catcher for six months. The blood gushing from the harpooned whales would attract deepwater ocean sharks, which surfaced to feed on them. Gimbel captured footage of these sharks for his 1971 documentary *Blue Water, White Death*. 'I can still hear the THUNK of the catchers' gun firing,' Valerie writes in *An Adventurous Life*, 'the heavy line spooling out towards the fleeing animal.'

She also explains:

If I lived a thousand years I would not be able to forget the cry of a dying whale. It goes through you and embeds in you. It's been speculated that the whale's mating call can cut through an entire ocean to another whale near another continent, but the sound of a whale dying can also cut through time. I can still hear the agony of the dying whales as their blood stained the water. I can hear its heart and soul. Not a beautiful sound like the song of a humpback but a deep, rumbling, pain-filled groan.

Whales are wonderful animals – peaceful and an important part of life on this planet – yet we slaughter them without remorse for a few tonnes of oil. Many had terrible wounds, they had fought and lost a battle for life against a metal ship with an exploding harpoon and a trained gunman to fire it.

They're intelligent too; Valerie cites footage of whales, entangled in ropes or nets, that swim towards a boat to ask for help. And footage of a dolphin ensnared in a fishing net approaching a diver, as if asking to cut it free. So many of the ocean's animals are not given enough credit. Sharks are so smart, she says, that she trained one to swim over a rock, with the perfect light behind it, for a photograph. 'It took less than an hour. I used fish scraps as a reward when the shark swam the right way.'

One astounding piece of footage in *Playing with Sharks* shows Valerie leaning off the back of their boat in South Australia to hand-feed a great white. 'There were three of them actually,' she recalls. 'But one of them had his head out of the water looking straight at me.' It could easily have leapt up and snatched her as she fed it and patted its nose. 'But I knew he wouldn't. He was a nice boy. Very polite.' She smiles. 'Sharks are like dogs, there are good and bad ones, they have different personalities.'

The most intelligent of all marine creatures, according to Valerie, is the octopus. 'I was diving by myself one day when I saw an octopus carrying a stone. She was building a wall. So I collected as many stones as I could and placed them down in front of her wall. She looked at me very directly, then carefully placed my stones on her wall. She was building around a hole. It was very impressive.'

Part of Valerie's tenacity can be attributed to her childhood. Her family had moved from Sydney to New Zealand for her father's work and, at twelve, she was one of thousands of children who contracted polio. Racked with terrible pain, unable to walk or move her arms over her head, she spent seven weeks in the polio ward of Wellington Hospital. Confined there, and isolated from her family, she underwent a highly effective – if agonising – treatment that involved warming the limbs with heat packs so they could be stretched by nurses. Thanks to this brutal approach, Valerie learned to walk again.

A group of Christians would visit the ward, bringing books: *Adventures of Huckleberry Finn*, *The Adventures of Tom Sawyer*, *Lorna Doone*. She spent every daylight hour in hospital with a book resting on a wooden holder; she would ask the nurses to turn the pages for her. These books opened the door to other lives, ones far more interesting than the one in which she found herself. 'I wanted to marry Tarzan or float down the Mississippi River with Huckleberry Finn. All I wanted to do from that moment on was to live an adventurous life.'

Moving back to Australia with her parents, at sixteen, was a step towards greater excitement. Settling in Burraneer Bay in Sydney's south, she learned to swim and snorkel, and then spearfish. It was at the St George Spearfishing Club that she fell in love with the best spearfisherman in Australia – Ron Taylor. For many months, despite doing everything she could think of to get his attention, the love was unrequited. It was when he started getting work for short underwater films that he began to seriously look at her. He realised the public were more interested in fish, especially dangerous ones like sharks, if a young blonde woman was swimming with them.

Life with Ron was the adventure she had been yearning for. Neither of them had much money but they had a dream and they believed in themselves. During the late 1960s and 1970s they saw a marine world they never knew existed and one they will never forget. 'We were two of the few people to see the reef in all its glory,' she recalls. 'The reef was a different place from what it is today. Fish life clouded the water or watched from small coral caves. It was a kaleidoscope of movement and colour.'

In 1967 she and Ron had the great good fortune of being part of a large six-month expedition to the Great Barrier Reef. It was led by a wealthy Belgian aristocrat and aspiring filmmaker, Pierre Dubuisson, who had been inspired by the underwater scenes in the James Bond film *Thunderball*. 'It was an aquatic empire the likes of which I had not seen before, and which I have not seen since,' she writes. It was an explosion of life: eels, sharks, fish, sea snakes, reef sharks, manta rays. At one stage they were nose to nose with a pod of pilot whales. It was during that trip, she recalls, that she and Ron saw 'the entire cycle of life, from the smallest animal to the largest'. It was there that she started to appreciate the 'balance and delicate beauty of marine ecologies'. She writes:

> *The reef is still beautiful, but for me ... it's like a flower in the sun that has faded. It's a former glory lost to a modern world. Many fish, such as the Queensland grouper and Maori Wrasse, have been harvested into rarity, and other species have succumbed to overfishing, and the sharks to finning ... Perhaps I should be thankful for having the opportunity to see something that so few ever saw. That's not how I feel, though.*

It has been heartbreaking, she says, watching its depletion. 'Diving with sharks was like going back in time. We had entered a world unchanged for a million years, and survived to tell its tale. There used to be so many fish that Ron and I once had to wait for twenty minutes while a school of kingfish swam past because they were casting a shadow over us while Ron was filming.'

Spending so long under the waves has given her an acute appreciation of the abundance and preciousness of marine life. 'I've realised that for every insect or animal or bird on land there is an equivalent in the ocean. There is the butterfly fish, for example, which is the bird of the sea.'

Valerie's life reads like a witness statement on the devastating changes to the ocean in her lifetime and the impact humans have had on nature. She's watched permanent damage being done to the environment for sport or business. 'I wish the Russians would stop harvesting krill. There isn't one animal or bird in Antarctica that doesn't rely directly or indirectly on krill for survival. The Russians use it for chicken food, cattle food. They have a voracious appetite for it.'

It's dangerous, Valerie says, to think that the marine environment will endlessly replenish itself. 'To be successful, a farmer must reap and sow, but fishers simply reaped. No one is ensuring the fish will be there next year. You can't just keep harvesting. You eventually have to give back, or you'll lose one of our greatest assets.

'Marine animals are free for the taking but unless we change our ways one day there will be nothing left to take. We need marine sanctuaries, where humans don't take and destroy. We need our reefs to be protected, and the impact of mining, runoff and pollution to be taken seriously.'

Ron and Valerie's despair deepened as the years passed and they witnessed not only dying reefs and thinning populations of large fish, but fewer and fewer sea lions at some of their favourite haunts. Valerie was used to opposition when it came to protecting sharks, but was taken aback at the death threats they received when they tried to protect the sea lions. She and Ron suspected there were fishermen shooting them for sport. 'The selfishness and greed of some people astonishes me.'

What lifts her spirits, she says, is the passion of the next generation for marine conservation. She's thrilled to be passing on the baton. For many years, she has received fan mail from girls and young women from all over the world. She was hugely encouraged by the avid enthusiasm of young men and women in the audience when *Playing with Sharks* won a US documentary award. 'They all wanted to know what to do, how to be activists,' she says. 'They're just like me: they want to see animals that live in the ocean protected, to be able to live and love and breed in safety.'

Her deepest wish, she says, is for them to remain as steadfast and as dedicated as she has been. Working to save life in the world's oceans and reefs before it's too late. She would dearly love more people to understand that we are all part of the natural world and that we need to care for it and protect it before it is lost forever.

'I've probably run out of time to stop the decline, but younger people can do it,' she says. 'They hold the future of life in the oceans in their hands.'

CHAPTER 4

RUSTY MORAN AND THE VETERAN SURF PROJECT

Mavericks

~~~

TONY PEARCE IS living proof of the transformative power of surfing. Every Saturday morning, the 52-year-old army veteran drives for two hours to the New South Wales South Coast in his work van, which he's kitted out with a bed and a surfboard rack and, on the dashboard, some healing crystals.

Within minutes of arriving at Seven Mile Beach, 'Big Tony', as he is known, has changed into his wetsuit, grabbed his new fibreglass board and is out in the sea with a group of other surfers, catching the long rollers the beach is famous for. When the bigger waves throw them off, they dive under before resurfacing and letting out a few whoops of joy. Within seconds, they have clambered onto their boards again and are paddling back out into the onrushing foam. There's no way they will miss a precious moment of this weekly saltwater fix.

'I can't believe I've been missing out on this for so long,' Tony says as he emerges from the sea with a huge smile on his broad face. 'We call it stealth therapy because it creeps up and heals you while you're out having fun. The first wave I caught was better than my first line of speed.'

It may seem hard to believe but just a few years earlier, the former Australian Defence Force engineer's world had become very dark. Like countless other veterans, Tony had found himself homeless, unemployed and addicted to ice and amphetamines. The addiction, he says, led to him 'losing everything I had, everyone I loved'.

He reached rock bottom when he was involved in a police chase that led to him sitting on the side of the road in handcuffs. 'I realised if I kept going, I was going to end up either in jail or dead.'

The secret to his recovery was the Veteran Surf Project, a learn-to-surf school for military veterans and first responders with post-traumatic stress disorder and depression. The man behind it is former big wave surfer Rusty Moran, who noticed something remarkable when he set up his surf school near the small coastal town of Gerroa in 2017. Within a couple of months of weekly surfing lessons, some of his students, particularly defence force personnel from the nearby Navy base, reported that they had started to recover from the debilitating disorder.

'I was teaching a group of local doctors who came surfing to de-stress from their work,' Rusty recalls. 'One GP said she wished she could write a script for ten surf lessons for her patients instead of medication. So I thought, well, why not? Why don't I make this happen?'

A few years later, the Veteran Surf Project came into being and, in January 2021, Rusty began introducing veterans and first responders with PTSD to the great tonic of surfing.

'Surfing puts us into a flow state, because when we get on the wave we've got about five or ten seconds when we're fully focused and in the present moment, thinking of nothing else but being on that wave. It's meditative. Even just for a brief moment, but each moment accumulates over time. It rewires the brain eventually.'

Rusty slowly paddles out on his board, his salt-laden, shoulder-length hair slicked back off his face so he can keep a close watch over his students. 'Soldiers are trained the same way as surfers – to learn the skill set, then wait patiently and then burst into action, and get that big adrenaline hit. This similarity makes it a natural process for soldiers to tap into the healing benefits of surfing, and the ocean.'

Rusty has helped hundreds of students, including many first responders. One – known simply as 'Ankles', for the ankle monitor tucked discreetly under his wetsuit – credits Rusty's program for his freedom. When the former NSW police officer was charged with assault, resulting from cocaine abuse, he expected to be sentenced to prison for eighteen months. Instead, the judge was so impressed by the psychiatric report about his recovery within Rusty's program that he made specific orders for him to attend twice a week.

Rusty was nineteen when he began taking on the outer reefs of Hawaii with the likes of Ken Bradshaw and Mark Foo. It was the early 1990s and they were paid by sponsors to ride the world's biggest waves. They were the mavericks of the surfing world and thought they were immortal, tackling monster swells, often a kilometre or two from shore. This was in the days before competitive surfers had jet skis hovering close by in case anything went wrong. Whenever a leg rope broke and a surfer lost their board, it was considered uncool to accept any help while swimming back to shore. But then one day, things did go badly wrong.

Rusty was surfing next to Hawaiian big wave surfer Jim Broach when a giant set of waves – each the size of a five-storey building – broke right in front of them. Just before the first wave hit them, Rusty and Jim nodded at each other, then dived deep – about 9 metres down, as far as their leg ropes would let them. The violent turbulence of the first wave belted them hard. 'The first wave felt like being hit in the chest with a tractor tyre, emptying my lungs,' Rusty

~~~

'We call it stealth therapy because it creeps up and heals you while you're out having fun.'

~~~

recalls. He knew he had to stay calm by counting numbers and to fight the impulse to suck in air, knowing his lungs would fill with water.

Rusty surfaced, only to be confronted by five more gigantic waves. 'Each time I surfaced, I looked for Jim, but he was gone ... I couldn't see him at all.'

Three other surfing friends died that year. Rusty's turning point came a few months later, at the funeral of Mark Foo. 'Mark's friends were saying, "Well, he died doing what he loved", and I suddenly realised how crazy it was, what we were doing. I loved surfing, but I wasn't prepared to die doing it.' He flew home, proposed to his girlfriend, started a family, became a civil engineer, then a property developer, and finally worked out how to make a living doing what he most loved – teaching others to surf.

The backbone of the Veteran Surf Project is connecting with nature. 'Just having sand under their toes, and feeling the warm sun on their faces is therapeutic in itself,' Rusty says. 'Then throw in the adrenaline rush of the waves, and the physical workout and the camaraderie, and you've got something that really works.'

Stopping to reflect and savour each surf as a group is equally important. 'If you've ever noticed surfers after a surf, we like to loiter in the car park, trying to extend that refreshed feeling a little longer.' Rusty laughs. The veterans usually gather at a café at nearby Gerroa to brag about their rides and tease each other about wipeouts.

It can be hard for veterans to adjust to civilian life; they've been trained to be self-reliant, self-contained and not show any weakness, even though they desperately need to connect with others. They've forged strong bonds with each other in stressful situations. And when they leave the service – and lose the closeness of their unit – that's when things start falling apart. But here they can let their guard down and start swapping stories about their lives. One might admit he has trouble sleeping at night. Another to having a fight with his kids. 'The chat afterwards really helps,' Rusty says. 'They're usually feeling good because they have mastered a new skill, but it's also in chatting to the other vets that they realise they are not alone. Seeing others recover helps them recover too. They realise they are not a broken person, that there is hope.'

Tony's take on it is this: 'For the first time, I don't have to pretend to be anything other than what I am. VSP is like having instant brothers and sisters. We realised we are part of something bigger than ourselves, and that feels damn good.'

Tony was only seventeen when he joined the Australian Defence Force. He was proud of what he did – supporting frontline troops by building bridges and laying pipes for their water supply – but when he left, life came crashing down around him. Without the bonds of friendship he'd forged within the ADF, and without the safety net of a structured hierarchy and daily routine, he found himself struggling to build relationships, to hold down a job, or to control his spiralling drug addiction.

The culture of the ADF made it hard for him to adjust to civilian life. 'It's about being as stoic as possible – if you cracked, or showed any kind of vulnerability, the whole group were punished. Bed bashes were common. That's when, if you let everyone else down, they would burst into your room. You get woken up with a beating.'

And there was an enormous resistance to asking for help. 'A lot of military training is to be self-responsible, self-reliant. It's hard for military people to go and see a doctor,' Tony says. Many regard it as similar to reporting to the sergeant major. 'It's a very command-and-control, hierarchical structure. It's drummed into us that it's better to toughen up and shut up than reveal your vulnerabilities or show your defects.'

It wasn't until Tony was standing in the lift of the South Coast Private Hospital, which specialises in psychiatric illnesses, that life finally took a turn for the better. Each time he caught the lift, his gaze was drawn to an intriguing poster on the wall. It showed a kangaroo on a surfboard inside a roundel that read *Veteran Surf Project*. He was curious: the symbol for the Royal Australian Air Force was a kangaroo in a roundel, but this one looked like much more fun.

At first Tony was full of doubts. 'I kept thinking, I can't do this, I don't even have a wetsuit.' But a few weeks later, Tony found himself at Seven Mile Beach, standing knee-deep in salt water, clutching a surfboard, with a coterie of other veterans, police officers and first responders.

'Next thing I knew, a couple of these mates were pushing me onto the board and up onto a wave. It was a great moment in my life,' he remembers now. 'I had absolutely nothing in my head. Just a feeling of being completely in the moment, being aware of everything around me, and listening to my own breath. It didn't matter whether the waves were big or small, or which way the wind was blowing, I just had to get out there into it.'

During the course, Tony was able to reduce his anti-depressants and anti-anxiety medication to the bare minimum. 'The Veteran Surf Project is a big reason I am here today. This project literally saved my life. I was always resigned to the fact that I was going to die doing what I was doing. I thought I had no options. I wasn't planning on doing anything productive with my life because I didn't know I was going to be around for that long,' he says. 'This is the best therapy I've found by far. And better than any drug I've taken.'

Tony sits back and looks at the cobalt-blue water around him, stretched out as far as the eye can see. 'The thing about the ocean is that it will punish you if you don't pay attention to it. When you're in the ocean, no matter what your rank or station is in life, you are not the boss any longer. When I'm out on a wave, all the ordinary things that consume me fade away. You don't worry so much about whether you're rich or you're poor. Or what you have or don't have. Your brain slips into a different gear. You're in the present moment, and it's a wonderful place to be.'

Tony recently took part in a night surf with his VSP mates, and when he describes it, he does so with an intensity that borders on religious fervour. That night, they were treated to both a lunar eclipse and an underwater light show: the ocean was filled with bioluminescence, the magical glowing effect of millions of algae creating their own light in a chemical reaction, similar to the effect of fireflies or glow-worms. 'The waves and our wetsuits were glittering with this glowing light,' he says. 'It opened my eyes to the glories of nature.'

The long-term effects of learning to surf have been extraordinary for Tony. Not only is he holding down a job as a hearing technician, he's also healed the rift with his family. His voice quavers with emotion when he describes catching a wave with his nineteen-year-old son, or the joy it brings him being 'Pop' to his three grandchildren. 'What Rusty has done is provide a community for us. Of people who love the ocean. It's helped us all get back on our feet. It's better than any medicine you could ever find.'

What makes the program work is Rusty's understanding of how bleak life can be for veterans. He knows many of them are lost or in limbo when they leave the armed forces, where they've had mates and a clear purpose in life. 'Many are homeless. Many of them sleep under bridges,' he says. 'There are more than 7000 Australian veterans sleeping rough. It's a massive problem that hasn't really been dealt with.'

In a nearby café after their surf, Rusty's care for his students is touching. He pulls chairs up towards a long wooden table and sits quietly among them as they share videos of each other surfing. It's often here, having coffee together, that he sees the veterans' physical signs of PTSD. 'They sit with their back to the wall so they can see the entrance, and their head is turning to the left and the right, constantly scanning for bombers. It's impossible for them to truly relax and be at ease.' He shakes his head. 'One of our Iraq veterans noticed another guy who would close his eyes whenever he turned the ignition key to start his car. He gave him a slap on the back and said, "Yeah, I get it. I still do that sometimes too." It's an exhausting way to live, because the nervous system is stuck in fight-or-flight, and when the cortisol dries up, depression follows.'

It was no surprise to him that the Royal Commission into Defence and Veteran Suicide, launched in 2021, revealed that suicide rates for male veterans is almost 30 per cent higher than in the wider Australian male population. There were a staggering 1677 suicides between 1997 and 2021.

Australian Defence Force Chief Angus Campbell recently apologised unreservedly for the lack of veteran support. 'Our people deserve and should rightly expect the wellbeing support and care they need both during and after their service. I acknowledge that this has not always been the case and has tragically led to the death by suicide of some of our people.'

Rusty knows firsthand what it's like to live with PTSD. His father was only fourteen years old when he joined the Australian Merchant Navy and was dispatched to Papua New Guinea and the Solomon Islands during the Second World

War. His ship supplied the US Navy with munitions and took Japanese prisoners of war, and his crew were under fire. When he returned, he bore the weight of these experiences. He suffered PTSD for decades and turned, as many did, to alcohol.

Rusty grew up bracing himself against sudden bursts of anger from his father. 'It would come out of nowhere, just these huge rages, and leave us all reeling. I learned to be on high alert, to get out of his way. I was in fight-or-flight mode a lot of the time until Dad started going to Alcoholics Anonymous. He became an AA mentor for the last 45 years of his life and helped hundreds recover, and demonstrated the power of social support.'

Unlike his regular surf school, the VSP project is volunteer work for Rusty, but it is deeply satisfying. 'Nothing fills me with greater joy than receiving a text message that says something like *I was having a really crap week but that surf put such a smile on my face for the rest of the day,*' he says. Many of the participants stay in touch, texting or ringing him to say they are still doing well, months after finishing the course. And the program's success is not just anecdotal. Rusty's PhD thesis shows that his ten-week program has long-lasting beneficial impact in reducing the symptoms of PTSD, depression and anxiety.[*]

---

[*] Moran, R. et al., 'The long-term effect of surf therapy on posttraumatic stress, depression, and anxiety symptomology among current and former Australian Defence Force members – A nonrandomised controlled longitudinal study in a community setting, *Mental Health and Physical Activity*, October 2024, vol. 27, doi.org/10.1016/j.mhpa.2024.100629

One VSP participant, Derek Pyrah, found that he was left with deep emotional scars after active duty in Iraq. Derek was dispatched to the thick of the war zone in 2003, running the computer networks and cryptography. He was renowned for being lightning fast, but several months into his posting he began experiencing the debilitating symptoms of PTSD. To his despair, he found himself unable to carry out the simplest of tasks, such as setting up a user account. 'I'd go to do it and then my mind was a complete blank,' he recalls.

Worse, he found himself unable to contain his rage. 'I was suddenly arguing and fighting and telling my boss to get fucked and I've never done anything like that in my life. Everything was going weird. Everything was falling apart.'

When he returned home, Derek was a stranger to his family and friends. 'My wife and kids said to me years later that when I got off the plane it looked like me, but I didn't talk like me or walk like me. I was always a nice, caring person. But I became irritable, angry, snappy, confused, frustrated.'

He was unable to hold down a job, and was plagued by insomnia, nightmares and flashbacks about what happened in Iraq, which he still cannot talk about. But what made matters far worse was being 'pumped', as he puts it, with a 'rotating cocktail' of medications that included high doses of anticonvulsant, as well as anti-anxiety and antipsychotic medications: the heavy-duty kind used to treat schizophrenia and bipolar disorder.

He was unable to hold down
a job, and was plagued by
insomnia, nightmares and
flashbacks about what
happened in Iraq, which
he still cannot talk about.

The drugs turned him into a zombie, he says, and ruined his marriage. 'The psych meds were killing me. I wasn't able to express myself. I would basically just sit in a corner and drool. And the medication made me eat and eat. I was 40 kilograms overweight.' Derek stayed in a mental health hospital for a third of each year for nine years.

He eventually realised that to truly take stock of what had happened to him in Iraq, and to start getting his life back, he would need to get off the prescription drugs. With remarkable determination, he began weaning off them, slowly replacing them with far less harmful medicinal cannabis.

The withdrawal process was harrowing. At one point, Derek was curled up in a fetal position, sweating profusely, his skin itching. His brain, he says, felt as if it were 'racing around like rats in a cage and I had no idea how to stop it'. He was flirting with suicide on the day he drove past the sign for the Veteran Surf Project at Seven Mile Beach. Like Tony, he was intrigued by the kangaroo on a surfboard. 'I remember thinking, I'll just try giving one last thing a go.'

The first session was tough. 'I hadn't been to the beach since Iraq because the sand would trigger flashbacks. Over there it crept into everything: your clothes, your bags; it was in your eyes, in your teeth.' But he was drawn back to the beach for the second week, and it was then that a little miracle happened: he stood up on a surfboard.

'I will never forget it,' he says. 'It was such a small thing, but it was the most surreal experience. I was standing perfectly still. And the whole world was going past me. It just felt like the most wow moment in my life. There was nothing going through my head. It just fully sucked me in.

'Rusty taught me not just how to surf and get my balance on a board, how to pick a wave and how to catch a wave but also, most importantly, how to ground and connect and how to reduce my stress levels by breathing down in my belly and not in my chest. How to just slow everything down so that you focus on what you're doing. How to be in a flow state. It's a state where you appreciate everything around you because your brain has slowed down and is actually taking it all in. And there's nothing really to think about except being balanced on that board in the present moment.' His face softens at the recollection.

'It's the power of nature too – lying on the surfboard, surrounded by the white foam, aware of the rips and the tides, and, if you're lucky, you'll see something wonderful, like a pod of dolphins.'

Soon, surfing began to transform Derek's state of mind. Instead of flashbacks and paranoia, his mind was filled with images of the silvery bubbles that formed around his hand when he dived underwater. Or the joy, on placid days, of being absorbed by the big blue sky while he sat on his surfboard 'out the back', beyond the breakers, enjoying the quietness in the sun.

'Your pleasure orientation changes. Instead of thinking about what drugs I needed that day, I started thinking about the swell, the tides, the temperature, any bluebottle alerts, and how I was going to get that fantastic sensation of catching a wave again.

'I started feeling normal again. The hours after I surfed were the best hours all week. I started getting hooked on that calm but spacious and clear feeling you get after a surf. I realised it was partly a physical thing – the foam in the surf has a negative ionisation charge. You're getting grounded without even realising you're being grounded. It's partly the smell of the salt water, too, that's so good for you. It made me feel at peace, something I hadn't felt for a long time.'

Today Derek is healthier than he was in his twenties, and the surfing has brought him a great gift: the ability to be closer with his son and daughter. His son, from whom he was estranged, began staying over one night a week, then two, and now lives with him. 'We started going for a walk together, or going to the drag races, or going to movies,' Derek says. His daughter also wants him back in her life. 'Once I'd got off the psych meds and started surfing, my capacity as a human and a parent kept increasing. That's really my main aim in life now: to get better for my family, to be a better dad than I have been.

'The ocean sort of feels like it's holding me, healing me, making me a better person, and I wouldn't have known that if I hadn't met Rusty and started surfing.'

CHAPTER 5

DR CHELS MARSHALL

Malgun Woman

~~~~~

ON A COLD, gloomy day on a deserted beach just north of Urunga on the North Coast of New South Wales, First Nations scientist Dr Chels Marshall is building a small fire. With her teenage daughter Lacey by her side, she carefully arranges handfuls of dry ginger, bracken, banksia pods and driftwood that she's just plucked from the nearby bush. She leans in and blows the flickering flame alive.

The pair stand together, staring out to sea, as aromatic smoke drifts over them. Flanking them on each side are grey rocks that look like a pair of giant stranded dolphins.

'Giinagay gagaal, Giinagay yuggirr, gagu and jinda Warriirla Gaagala Ngaanya nyayagi,' they say together. ('Hello ocean, hello dolphins, my beautiful brothers and sisters in the east, in the sea, see me.') 'Before we greet the dolphins and move among them,' Chels explains, 'we need to cleanse ourselves with the smoke. This is our way of getting the dolphins to flourish, of looking after them. Because if you look after the ocean, it looks after you.'

If there is anyone in Australia in a position to know this, it's Chels. She is a woman who dances between two worlds, a bridge between traditional First Peoples' culture and modern marine science. Chels's family has called Gumbaynggirr – a glorious 120-kilometre parcel of beaches, rivers and estuaries, bordered by the Great Dividing Range, between the Clarence and the Nambucca rivers – home for countless years. 'Our family has been here for a long time. My great-grandmother was cremated here in the last traditional tree burial, and our family has survived here through the droughts and bushfires and floods and colonisation. We were here when this coast was formed,' she says. 'Long, long before colonisation.'

Gumbaynggirr women were astoundingly good fishers who would sing in dolphins to assist them. They held prestigious Malgun status. Malgun women were the high priestesses of fishing, chosen from a young age, who had part of their little finger removed as a sign of their vocation. 'The early colonists thought it was a misogynistic thing, that they were marked for marriage,' Chels says, 'but it was more a status symbol.'

These expert fisherwomen saved the first settlers from starvation by bringing them gifts from the sea – baskets brimming with flathead, bream, whiting and octopus. 'They were so respected that one of the first pieces of legislation in the colony was to respect the fishing equipment of the local Gadigal Aboriginal women. Anyone who stole or damaged their fishing gear was flogged.' Chels lights up as she tells this story. She loves sharing it with First Nations girls.

Chels grew up on Country not far from here, steeped in First Nations teachings, in a beach shack built out of tin, driftwood and timber from marine debris on the Nambucca River. Her father, Okie, who worked in the local sawmill and played for the local football team, caught mackerel and snapper. Her mother, Frances, taught Chels and her siblings, including her late brother Lustin, how to collect pipis, fish for mullet and forage in the bush for warrigal greens, or wild spinach. 'There was always an abundance of food, plenty to share with friends who needed it,' she says.

Just as their parents had, and their parents before them, Okie and Frances taught their children how to understand the ocean and to care for its creatures. As soon as she could walk, Chels was learning how to read the tides, and the winds, and the behaviour of marine life, with as much – if not more – accuracy than the Bureau of Meteorology. 'My family all knew the ocean intimately and had a great respect for it. They used Indigenous knowledge to look after it with great care. We have been fishing here for thousands of years, so it was in our interests to look after the ocean,' she says.

They were in tune with the seasons and worked with them to their advantage. Her father and uncles fished with great finesse, spearing off the rock platforms or casting handmade nets into the ocean when the fish were at their fattest, and most nutritious. That way, they did not need to overfish. 'They would wait for the southerly wind to blow, just after the butterflies arrived. That's when they knew the mullet would be leaving the estuary and start migrating out to the ocean. They would get their spears and nets out.'

They cooked crabs and fish over coals and soup made with curry powders. They'd mince pipis and freeze them so they could prepare pipi soup and pipi fritters. 'We didn't have much money to spend at the supermarket, but we always knew what to gather and pick and when. We knew where to get the best fish, and when. We knew the personalities of the fish and the birds.'

One of the ways First Nations People look after the sea is through their totem system. A family or mob's connection to a particular marine animal is deeply personal, and ironclad. 'We protect our totem as if they are kin,' Chels says. 'Your totem could be the pelican, the black bream, a shark, a black swan, a stingray or a turtle. You become the expert on your totem and help educate others about its role and function in

~~~

Chels is a woman who dances between two worlds, a bridge between traditional First Peoples' culture and modern marine science.

~~~

the environment.' You'd never harm or kill your totem; your main function would be to help it thrive.

Her mother's totem, passed on to her, was the yugirr, or dolphin, highly respected as elders in the ocean. 'They are regarded as equal to humans, and they like helping us with our fishing,' she explains. 'There is a story of one of my uncles walking along the beach, spearing fish, and he was having trouble, and a dolphin would herd the fish in towards him so he could catch them. It was teamwork. He would throw the fish back to the dolphin so it was a reciprocal thing.'

It seems only natural that she too would have a special affinity with the yugirr. As a girl, she learned that if she dived under the waves and watched them closely, and listened for long enough, she could tune in to their clicks and squeals. 'They're very social. They talk to each other a lot about where they're going and what the other pods are doing, where they caught a heap of fish the week before, or where their favourite fishing spots are. It's just like any other language – once you tune in to it, you can start to understand them.' She could tell if they were distressed or if they were happy and chatty.

'The mothers are incredibly protective. They spend a lot of time talking to their little ones, warning them where not to go, to stay away from the sand bars, stay away from this particular shark or that one. They're very playful too – they often play with sponges and throw them around and play chasey.'

She learned to get their attention, or warn them of danger, by clapping rocks together under the water. One of the most thrilling moments of her childhood was when, as Chels was looking after her younger cousins at the water's edge, a mother dolphin herded her calves towards her to watch while she went fishing. 'I was literally babysitting little dolphins.'

Their intelligence borders on telepathic, Chels explains, as we keep an eye on the surface, looking for telltale signs in the water. 'They communicate with ultrasonic signals, or sound, they emit to each other through a melon, a fatty tissue at the top of their head. I can hear them, I can feel them, I can sense them,' she says. 'I was walking along the water recently with Lacey and I said to her, "I can feel the family coming through." She was sceptical, she was laughing and not too sure whether to believe me or not, but I ended up calling them in and, next thing we knew, they had appeared right in front of her. It just blew her mind.'

Lacey, listening in, smiles shyly. She's striking – willowy and graceful – and dreams of joining the Bangarra Dance Theatre in Sydney. Chels, just as unassuming, likes to be as inconspicuous as possible. In her trademark loose, natural-coloured T-shirt and trousers, she almost blends into the natural environment around her.

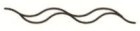

The natural saltwater lifestyle of Chels's childhood has long disappeared; their shack has gone and her parents have passed away. But the desire to preserve and protect the ocean

~~~

'Why wouldn't you want to use the knowledge that has been tried and tested for over 65,000 years?'

~~~

as a First Nations Knowledge Keeper has become a central force of her life.

Her parents had to leave school in Grade Five to go to work, but they instilled in their daughter the importance of education. Chels became a First Nations trailblazer. She topped her classes at school and won a traineeship at the National Parks and Wildlife Service as a ranger, one of the first Indigenous people to do so.

Two degrees, a Master of Marine Science and a PhD, soon followed and, today, Chels is an expert in sea management. She has discussed climate change with world leaders, like President Macron of France, and advises the CSIRO and the Commonwealth Department of Environment about First Nations marine science. By this she means the sophisticated ecological knowledge that Aboriginal and Torres Strait Islander people have been using for thousands of years, much of which has been lost, hidden or forgotten since colonisation.

'Why wouldn't you want to use this knowledge?' she asks calmly. 'After all, we've got nothing to lose, and everything to gain.' The potential demise of the environment and the species within it prompt the question: 'Should we try switching it up a bit and using the knowledge that has been tried and tested for over 65,000 years?'

Spending time with Chels and Lacey is like seeing the world with new eyes, or with 'Indigenous glasses', as Chels puts it. As she talks, she is scanning the horizon, where the ocean meets the sky. Although dolphins don't appear in the stormy sea, she has a strong sense they are close by. 'There's a pod of two or three of them out there, probably a mother and her babies,' she says.

Then, far out to sea, she spots the dark, arched backs and spouts of humpback whales. 'When the whales started migrating we used to signal to our mob all the way up and down the coast with message sticks and fire sticks – that was our form of a telephone, or a text message.' She leans in to blow the flames a little more. 'These ones are heading south now they've had their babies. There are storms out to sea, and the snapper are out, so that attracts the bull sharks.' If there is a mother dolphin out there, she'd be busy teaching her babies where to swim, to avoid being eaten by the sharks, she says.

Seeing things through Chels's eyes gives a much more expansive view of the world. 'Western science is so narrow in comparison to Indigenous science and ideology. For instance we [the Gumbaynggirr] have more than four seasons; being this close to the equator, the seasons are variable and are not as clear-cut as in the Northern Hemisphere.

'Our knowledge is holistic. It reaches from the depths of the ocean right up to the stars and the constellations.' She gestures to the sky. 'The white star of Venus, or the red star of Mars were seasonal indicators; they'd tell us that the yellow-breasted robin would be on the way, or a particular tree was about to blossom.'

Earlier, she and Lacey were sitting on a timber seat over-looking Muttonbird Island Nature Reserve, at the north end of Coffs Harbour. It was a Sunday morning, and the promenade was full: families walking dogs and pushing children in strollers, couples jogging, and older folk reading the newspapers and chatting in the sun at the kiosk. It's a wonderful place for a swim or a walk, or to have coffee with friends, but for Chels and Lacey, it has a deeper meaning. In their eyes, the island and harbour are traversed with energy lines and dreaming tracks of the creation ancestors. Every rock or shell – every sweep of the headland – is imbued with a spiritual meaning. The creation of the landscape, Chels explains – the mountains, rivers, stone formations – everything took place 'in a time none of us would have comprehension of; in time and scale it is immortal'.

One of the many ingenious ways First Nations People have looked after the sea around us is to have protected zones enshrined into their lore and songlines. Many of the protected areas we have today have been protected in Indigenous culture for centuries. Stories imbued with highly practical ways of looking after the ecosystem were told from one generation to the next. She points to Muttonbird Island, in front of her, as an example. 'The island is guarded by Giidan, the giant moonman.' Only certain people from the right families and section of the community could go to the island and then only at certain times and tides, she explains. Everyone else was banned. If the rules were broken, tidal waves, rips and floods would follow.

'It meant visitation was restricted, and that everybody couldn't just march onto the island and help themselves to the mutton birds or eggs and other resources there. This was the way we made sure the mutton birds were not over-harvested, and balance and harmony prevailed so there was always enough to eat in the community.'

Today, First Nations People are preserving special and protected areas not just through stories but through native title as well. 'More than 80 per cent of native title land is bio banks that make up Australia's national reserve system, which protects biodiversity and threatened species,' Chels says. 'Native title is actually helping Australia reach our biodiversity and climate targets.'

Blue Mud Bay in the Northern Territory, to the east of Darwin native title, is a classic example. Commercial fishers need permission from the Traditional Owners before they can enter the sea country. As a result, says Chels, barramundi, mud crabs and trepang (sea cucumber) are finally being fished sustainably and are out of danger of being overfished.

In First Nations thinking, everything is connected. The health of the ocean is inextricably entwined with the health of First Peoples. 'Our demise is commensurate to the demise of the sea creatures. If the country is sick, we are sick,' she says,

~~~

**Every rock or shell – every
sweep of the headland – is
imbued with a spiritual
meaning.**

~~~

shaking her head sadly. 'It's no coincidence that when colonisers removed Aboriginal people from the land it also resulted in the dramatic depletion of species and the mismanagement of Country. That's why we have so many problems today. The issues around fire and flood are perfect examples.'

Despite despairing over the regular headlines of coral bleaching and declining marine species populations, Chels remains encouraged by Western marine scientists who are beginning to listen to, and incorporate, Indigenous ways of looking after the sea. There is no doubt our appreciation of First Nations science and sea and land management has grown over the last decade. 'The early settlers thought Australia was this beautiful natural park, that it was just naturally well maintained, with very little undergrowth between tall trees and verdant grass,' she says. 'But it was actually the work of our people. We kept the land, the animals, the wildlife, in a pristine condition with balance and harmony in a somewhat symbiotic relationship.'

Bruce Pascoe's *Dark Emu* and Bill Gammage's *The Greatest Estate on Earth* both broke new ground, presenting First Peoples in a new light. Both Pascoe and Gammage wrote that First Nations People were far more than hunters and gatherers. They sowed and rotated crops, ground grain, baked bread, trapped fish, built stone homes and managed bushfires with great skill by burning back the undergrowth.

Our education system has also recognised that truth telling is important, she says. Through hard work and lots of study, Chels has created a good life – she owns a home nearby, built of recycled windows and doors, surrounded by paperbark trees, and a hinterland property where she and her younger brother grow native food. But many others have not been so lucky. European settlement had a devastating effect on the First Peoples of the Mid North Coast. Their lands were cleared and fenced, and thousands were forced to live in makeshift shanty towns on the fringes. They were subjected to massacres, child removal, and being moved en masse to missions. European diseases such as smallpox also decimated the community.

Chels takes a deep breath before talking about the entrenched racism her parents experienced. 'They were made to walk on different sides of the road. They went to missionary school rather than the mainstream school, and went to different shops. They were called abos, n***s and coconuts.' Her aunt was part of the Stolen Generation, taken from her parents and sent to Sydney to work as a servant in a wealthy family. She's witnessed family members who have lost their rights to fish and live where their mob have lived for generations. What keeps her going, she says, is the inherent strength of her people. 'We have survived the last 238 years, and our culture will continue to survive. We are highly resilient peoples, we are innovative and we think a bit differently to most,' she says.

Her focus over the next few years will be keeping Indigenous knowledge alive by remapping the songlines of cetaceans. By this, she means the stories, told through ceremonial dance and song, art and oral histories, about the journeys of marine life. These stories are vessels that contain information about landmarks such as river mouths, rocks, tides, the sky, the stars and trees, as well as the seasons.

'We've always done this – embedded our knowledge about marine life in song and dance, by remembering and learning and then practising – but a lot of it has been sleeping. Now it is time to wake it up and take our place in Country.' She takes a long breath, looking intently towards the horizon. 'We're hoping to empower our mob to bring it back, so that we can all take better care of the ocean.'

The federal government is starting to pay attention to the importance of these ancient stories, and has recently funded a $300,000 study into Indigenous songlines to protect our whales and dolphins.

The ocean, meanwhile, remains Chels's personal sanctuary. Her feet naturally gravitate towards the shore not far from her home whenever she is troubled or anxious or confused. 'I love the fact that the ocean is a life entity in itself. It decides what it wants to do, and where it wants to go. Some days it is volatile, other times it is calm and inviting.'

As she speaks, a giant sea eagle hovers, circles and swoops down onto the shoreline, landing at her daughter's feet. She, too, finds strength within the ocean. 'Whenever I feel nervous before I have to get up and perform,' Lacey says, 'I repeat to myself, "I am a strong Gumbaynggirr ocean woman."'

Chels looks contemplative. She can't talk much longer – she wants to pick some native food on her property before nightfall – and hurries away, disappearing into the long shadows on the beach.

CHAPTER 6

JESSICA WATSON

Liquid Mountains

~~~

JESSICA WATSON WAS sixteen years old when she set out from her home town of Mooloolaba on Queensland's Sunshine Coast to sail around the world, solo and unassisted. Ahead lay a 211-day journey across some of the most remote and dangerous stretches of ocean on the planet.

It started less than perfectly. Her ability to stay positive during tough times was tested on her very first night at sea. Lying in her bunk, about 15 nautical miles away from Stradbroke Island, Jessica was awoken by the terrifying sound of her little boat, *Ella's Pink Lady*, colliding with a

63,000-tonne bulk carrier, *Silver Yang*. 'I remember looking up, and the carrier was so large the night stars were obscured by its giant steel walls.'

There was damage to the mast of her boat, but the toughest part was remaining dignified as she sailed into the Gold Coast in front of the crowds and the waiting media. She knew the accident would confirm the worst fears of those who doubted the wisdom of letting a sixteen-year-old girl set off on her own around the world.

As she stood in front of the microphones, her stalwart manager Andrew Fraser by her side, she held her head high. Yes, she admitted, she had made a mistake by forgetting to set the alarms that would alert her to approaching ships. But she would not let it get the better of her. The trip would continue.

From that point on, she became a household name.

Like most sailors who want to test their abilities, Jessica was drawn, as if by a siren's song, to the Southern Ocean, the body of water beneath Australia, South America and Africa, encircling Antarctica. It's the second smallest of our oceans, but throws up monstrous waves and wind. 'It's this notorious, stupid place with big grey waves and ferocious storms,' she says.

What amazed her was how *fast* the water was moving. 'The waves are incredibly powerful because they run the whole way around the world and they are not stopped by land.' Sailing across the Southern Ocean in her little boat made her feel 'thrillingly alive'. 'It was similar to stepping out into a thunderstorm, but multiplied by about a hundred.'

She learned to trust *Ella's Pink Lady* as much as her own natural abilities. She talked to her yacht, urging it on as it pitched and rolled in the cold, remote seas. She turned its tiny size into an asset: it enabled her to open her arms to the raw power of the Southern Ocean.

By the time she'd spent several months at sea, she had learned to read the weather by paying attention to the surface of the ocean, and by watching the sky, as much as studying the synoptic charts. 'You start to work it out. You see this bad weather coming because there are these subtle changes in the way the water is moving.'

The most terrifying moments were when a monster wave was approaching. 'You'd hear it roaring like a train in the distance,' she recalls. 'You knew that in a few minutes it was going to come thundering towards you.' She would quickly strap herself in, down below deck, in her life jacket, her knees shaking, her guts churning. 'Sailors don't stand on the foredeck in front of the boat in a 30-knot wind,' she says. 'That's just for the movies. When a ferocious storm arrives, you've only got one thought in mind: survival.'

In one of the storms she faced, in the South Atlantic Ocean, she battled waves that were almost 30 metres high – the size of apartment blocks. Such was the ferocity of the gale that her Sparkman & Stephens 34 – one of the safest, toughest little sailing boats in the world – was knocked down several times, once to the point where her boat was almost 3 metres underwater. Strapped into her life jacket below deck, the teenager gritted her teeth and held on until the storm had passed, ringing her terrified parents on the satellite phone every few hours to let them know she was still alive. She then continued on, navigating thousands of nautical miles across the world's oceans without stopping once.

On a solo voyage, you can't ever completely unwind. Jessica was almost always on deck, and on guard, always on alert for unpredictable weather – from eerie fogs to 40-knot gales to the deeply frustrating 'doldrums' as she neared the equator, where there was no breeze for days.

Being out on such vast, remote stretches of salt water with no one else to rely on taught her a great deal about self-reliance. In fact, a large part of the trip was not so much the physical act of sailing as it was learning how to cope with tough times. 'Most of the time I was fine but then, *boom*, out of nowhere I'd really want someone to come and give me a hug.' As she says this, perched at an outdoor table of a Melbourne café, it's suddenly apparent how slight her frame is. She learned to combat loneliness by staying busy with small tasks, keeping her yacht shipshape, putting music on, or ringing family and friends via the satellite phone.

She found strength she did not know existed. 'I realised it was possible to feel really anxious and worried – with no sleep, and terrified – but also incredibly strong,' she says.

~~~

'I remember looking up, and the carrier was so large the night stars were obscured by its giant steel walls.'

~~~

'I realised courage is not about not being afraid; it's about keeping going when you are terrified.'

It helped that all around her was the consoling and sustaining beauty of the ocean. 'The ocean is so mysterious, and it's always changing. It never ceases to fascinate me,' she says. Her online blog recorded its splendour: the sight of the stars at night, reflected in the ocean like a mirror; whales breaching; the phosphorescent glow of hundreds of jellyfish rising to the surface from the depths below. After she'd endured a fierce storm, she always found it uplifting to see a pod of dolphins leap beside her yacht, looking directly at her. 'I'm sure they were checking that I was okay,' she says.

It seems hard to believe now, but Jessica was afraid of the water as a girl. It was only when her older sister and cousins were leaping into the swimming pool that she finally decided to take the plunge herself. 'I got tired of sitting by the side of the pool watching them have fun,' she recalls.

Her family were adventurous; they went camping or took four-wheel drive trips during the school holidays. Learning to sail was a family activity. When she was in Grade Four, her parents enrolled her in a sailing club at nearby Southport. As with swimming, she was apprehensive – at first. 'I spent a lot of time on the beach and on the shore watching the others out there having fun before I plucked up the courage to do it myself.'

Her love of sailing deepened when her parents bought a 52-foot motorboat. It was supposed to be for a family holiday, for a month or two, but they ended up cruising up and down the eastern coast for five and a half years, during which time they fixed almost every part of the boat.

School was by correspondence, guided by her mother. 'They were – and still are – such original thinkers,' Jessica says of her parents. 'They planted the seed that you can live an adventurous life.' They stopped at islands where they were the only boat. The day would unfold with snorkelling, swimming, collecting shells, exploring beaches, gullies and waterways and lighthouses. 'My parents gave me self-confidence, self-belief, and helped me understand that ordinary people could do extraordinary things. I've got a lot to be thankful for. That positive approach set me up for life.'

On weekend sailing adventures with her older sister Emily and younger siblings Hannah and Tom, she learned how to get herself out of any trouble. There were no mobile phones. She learned to trust her instincts. 'Bad things can happen, but bad things can happen anywhere and wrapping us in cottonwool was not necessarily going to keep us safe. Mum and Dad made a deliberate choice to let us have space to explore and they trusted us to do the right thing.'

When Jessica was eight, soon after she began sailing on the Gold Coast, her mother gave her *Lionheart*, the

~~~

'My parents gave me
self-confidence, self-belief,
and helped me understand
that ordinary people could
do extraordinary things.'

~~~

biography of Jesse Martin, who, at eighteen, had become the youngest person to sail solo, nonstop and unassisted, around the world. She read it from cover to cover several times, her imagination seized by the teenager's bravery, all the while secretly wondering if she could attempt something similar.

She began by making small offshore trips with her older sister on the Sunshine Coast. During the course of one, when she was thirteen, she experienced a defining moment. Out on a 23-foot yacht, she, Emily and a fifteen-year-old family friend, Nick, got stuck in a huge swell. When Nick and Emily both became unwell, Jessica was the only one who could still sail. 'Up until then, I would have been the first person to go to pieces in a situation like this, but I suddenly had to take matters into my own hands,' she recalls. 'I was drenched and exhausted, but I had to start making decisions myself.' She took the tiller and guided the yacht slowly out of the storm and into calmer waters. 'I realised I could influence things myself, with my own actions. It was a matter of building up confidence in myself.'

Once she had overcome her fears, she was hooked. 'I would rather be sailing than anywhere else in the world. I love the challenge of making my own decisions and overcoming the problems thrown at me. When I am on the water, reefing a sail or tacking in response to the wind and the waves, everything becomes very simple.'

As her dream of sailing around the world grew, she became a sponge, spending her free time asking other sailors for advice. Many of them told her the same thing: good sailors need to be as strong mentally as they are physically. They also told her she needed to be a good all-rounder who could do everything herself: cooking, electrical repairs, rigging, plumbing, watching the weather.

As her confidence grew, she took on more adventurous trips, crewing on professional yachts around New Zealand and Vanuatu. By the time she'd set out to sail around the world, she'd clocked up more than 10,000 nautical miles on the open water. She buckled down and completed courses in engine maintenance and meteorology.

She never felt judged or inadequate because she was a teenage girl. Sailing may be a male-dominated sport but Jessica said she felt 'nothing but extraordinary support from so many old blokes. I've never felt anything but totally protected.' As seasoned adventurer Don McIntyre, who was a great supporter and helped her buy a yacht for the trip, put it: 'She hasn't been pulled out of the bedroom, playing with dolls, and plonked on a boat. Age isn't relevant here. It's who she is, what she is, and what's driving her.'

One of the secrets of her success is positive thinking. At home in her room, she pinned up images of the notoriously vast, remote and treacherous Southern Ocean, and visualised herself tackling 'liquid mountains', as she called the biggest swells. She'd trained with a psychologist in the basics of cognitive behavioural therapy before she left the shore. 'Mainly it's about stopping your mind catastrophising,' she says.

'It's about being disciplined and taming your mind – and just seeing things for what they are, and accepting that it will eventually change, rather than blowing it out of proportion.'

So is there a specific example of how this helped her sail around the world? 'There were days on the trip when I was just miserable, so it was helpful to talk to myself positively. I knew I wasn't depressed. It was just the physical situation: I was cold and wet and a bit lonely, and that it would be different tomorrow.'

There was some fierce criticism of her parents, for allowing a teenage girl to attempt such a feat, but before she left, they, and her mentors, made sure Jessica had state-of-the-art communications equipment on board. She had two handheld satellite phones – one for everyday use and the other for an emergency grab bag if she ever had to abandon ship. She had internet connection through a small satellite dome on the stern, enabling her to update her blog and send video clips, photos and emails. There was also a high-frequency radio for prearranged radio link-ups. And, of course, there was a tracker fitted on the boat, sending constant signals to the appropriate people – which would sound an alarm if there were any ships approaching.

As she began the final leg of her seven-month trip, she felt like the world was watching – and willing her on. Arriving in Sydney Harbour was bittersweet. As thrilling as it was to finally return, part of her would miss the simplicity of being out in the wind and the waves, surrounded by salt water as far as her eyes could see. The stillness and the silence she'd experienced, as well as a respect for the vastness of the ocean, and its raw and unpredictable nature, have remained with her ever since.

The solo trip was an extraordinary feat that earned her an Order of Australia and, more than a decade later, she remains one of our greatest role models for the youth of Australia. Few will forget the jubilation of her return in May 2010. A flotilla of yachts and boats surged out to greet her with cheers and horns, almost swamping her tiny yacht. As she moored at the Opera House and stepped into the arms of her waiting parents, the crowd went wild.

'Our Jess', as she quickly became known, endeared herself even more when, at her glittering reception, she firmly disagreed with the prime minister, Kevin Rudd, that she was a new national hero. 'I don't consider myself a hero,' she told the packed forecourt. 'I'm just an ordinary girl who had a dream, believed in it, and worked hard.'

Still, she did prove that day that anything was possible. In the best-selling book she wrote after the trip, *True Spirit*, and more recently, in the movie adaptation, she explains that her success was due to meticulous preparation – both physically and psychologically. 'I knew I was a young girl and that I didn't have the physical strength of a fully grown man, so I had to work out ways that suited me and my body,' she wrote. 'To me, sailing is not about strength, it is about knowledge.'

Several years ago, Jessica completed an MBA in business management, which she uses in her role at the international accounting firm Deloitte. With a small team, she helps companies adapt to the explosion of new technology. 'Sometimes clients are surprised to see "that sailor girl" sitting at the board table in such a highly corporate environment, but on the whole I fit right in. I really love the work, and the team,' she says.

Such is the power of her profile and story that she is still in demand as a motivational speaker. She speaks to everyone from schoolchildren to corporate high flyers. Their most common questions haven't changed: How did you manage your fears during the huge seas? How high were the waves? Did you see any sharks? How did you manage the yacht at night on your own? But what most people don't realise, as they listen to her story, is that, since then, Jessica has faced something far more challenging than the monstrous waves of her circumnavigation.

'It's taken far more out of me, far more courage, to go on without Cam,' she says.

Cam was Cameron Dale, a fellow sailor she fell in love with a year after her circumnavigation and with whom she had been 'inextricably entwined' since then. They met on the 2011 Sydney to Hobart Yacht Race; Jessica was the skipper of the youngest crew to compete, and Cam was one of her crew members. 'I remember thinking, Whoa, who is *this*? And trying to hide how much I was taken by him,' she says.

They were both feisty, and initially clashed a lot. Cam thought the crew should rest when the weather was calm, but Jessica thought it was more important they maintain the ship while they had the chance. They saw a mediator after the trip to sort out their differences. Detached from the race, and duty, romance blossomed. After a long-distance relationship, Jessica moved down from the Sunshine Coast to be with Cam in Melbourne.

Both had driven natures – there's only a tiny coterie who can say they have sailed solo around the world as a teenager or competed in the notoriously dangerous Sydney to Hobart Yacht Race – but sailing was never a professional pursuit for either of them. 'I didn't need to prove myself,' Jessica says. 'I'm not an Olympic-style racing sailor.' Both she and Cam adored just being out on the ocean. It's remained a passion, a hobby. They were happiest when they were 'mucking about' on Port Phillip Bay. 'There is something so utterly beautiful about the feeling of power of a boat under sail. There's nothing like it in the world,' Jessica says.

She and Cam were planning a life together, a family. 'We were looking forward to taking our baby out on a yacht with us.' But in September 2021 all their plans – and Jessica's world – came crashing down.

'He'd been complaining about not feeling well for quite a while, but he was always loath to see a doctor, and then during COVID the consultations were via telehealth, which didn't help,' she says. They were on the Gold Coast, as technical consultants for Jessica's Netflix film, when Cam suddenly felt 'incredibly unwell'. He had a throbbing headache, nausea and pins and needles in his fingers. 'He was saying, "This doesn't feel like something normal, this feels really bad."'

When they realised he was having a minor stroke, he was rushed to the nearest hospital. They discovered he had undiagnosed high blood pressure. Another stroke in hospital, this time major, proved fatal. He was 29, and otherwise in good health, with no underlying health issues.

Loving – and then losing – Cam has changed Jessica irrevocably. She has a measured, reserved manner but, despite the winter sunshine pouring into the café around her, the sense of loss is searing. Still, there is a palpable sense of relief when the conversation turns away from sailing and towards him. She's been asked to talk about her circumnavigation many times, but her story doesn't end there. 'Sometimes I feel like a musician who is being asked to sing the same song again and again. Yet there has been a whole life I've spent with Cam since then. I don't want people to think my life is happily ever after. It's not.' To not talk about him, to not include him in her story, she says, 'is not right'.

She's adjusting to the new reality, that he is no longer by her side. 'I still buy too much bread, forgetting that he's not there to eat half of it.' She thinks about him when she goes home at night, when she instinctively wants to share something funny that happened in the office that day. 'We were together for so long that who I am and the life we had together can't be separated.'

She's even developed mannerisms that are like his. 'It's quite strange, since he's passed away I've become interested in sailing equipment, and how things work, the way he used to be. I even like drinking beer.'

Grief is physical, she says. At various times, sometimes all at once, there will be a terrible ache in her chest, a sickness in the stomach, sudden bursts of tears. Sometimes this frightens her, especially the heart palpitations and panic attacks. Worse, though, is the discombobulation of no longer having a future together. She'd become accustomed to seeing the world through Cam's eyes, and hearing his take on things. Without his views, his opinions, his anecdotes about the day, life seemed flat and dull. At rock bottom – which she doesn't like to dwell on for more than a couple of seconds – life seemed pointless. 'The pain was so bad that I just didn't want to exist in a world where Cam wasn't with me. I don't think I realised you could be in so much pain until he passed away,' she says. 'I just wanted the pain to end.'

What pulled her out of the depths was being near what had sparked the most joy in her life: the ocean. Being near it, being able to see it, smell it and touch it has helped heal her, calm her. When she's sailing, she is grateful to be alive.

During the traumatic weeks of visiting Cam in hospital after he'd suffered his first stroke, the mere act of gazing at the ocean was a consolation. 'I remember looking out the car window on the way to the hospital and stopping to look at the ocean. It had never looked so beautiful, the way the late afternoon sun was reflecting on the choppy deep blue surface. I couldn't believe I was still able to appreciate the beauty of nature when I was in so much pain,' she says.

Getting out on the water has been the greatest balm since losing him. Her friends instinctively rallied around her. 'They are just amazing support. They'll ring me up to say they need a hand fixing something, and could I come on down and check it out? I think some of the time it's just an excuse to get me out on the water.'

And once she's out on the ocean, she lets the tears flow.

'I've always found the ocean the best way to get my bearings, but it's definitely amplified in the last year and a half since I've lost Cam,' she says. 'It's been a real solace.' Mostly, it's where she feels closest to him. 'When I'm out on the water, with the wind on my face, when I see the clouds, when I see the sunlight dancing on the water, my thoughts are always of him.' She looks down at her plate. 'Sometimes it feels like he is so close to me that I could almost reach out and touch him when I'm out on the deck.'

Since Cam's death she has gradually found ways to enjoy her life again – hard work, being fit, doing yoga, being with family and friends. But it is sailing that has given her the most powerful desire to be alive. Being immersed in the wind and waves, especially with Cam's friends, is the most powerful antidote to despair, and the best way to keep her head in order.

~~~

**'Life is so precious, so
fleeting ... Throw yourself
into it. Life is nothing
but a daring adventure.
Have big dreams.'**

~~~

Cam's death brought her face to face with the truth of how fragile life is. 'Life is so precious, so fleeting. Young people often ask my advice, and what I say to them is: embrace life. Throw yourself into it. Life is nothing but a daring adventure. Have big dreams.'

It's also taught her about the power of love. 'It's the simple realisation that you don't ever have to move on. You can go on to live a great life. But it doesn't mean you forget the person. They're not here physically with you to talk to, to touch, but they are in your memories, in the world, in your heart. And there's no denying that's real. They are part of you. You just have to learn to love them in a different way.'

CHAPTER 7

YUSRA METWALLY

Burkini Babe

~

YUSRA METWALLY KNOWS exactly how it feels to be excluded from mainstream beaches. As a devout Muslim, she has always been aware of Sydney's quiet underbelly of racism. Despite this, she was still deeply shocked when, one evening in December 2005, she sat down to watch the evening news about a race riot at her favourite place to swim: Cronulla Beach.

Yusra, her siblings and her parents, who had emigrated to Sydney from Egypt when she was nine, sat in horrified silence as the bulletin showed a mob of more than 5000 angry

Anglo-Australians – mainly young men without shirts – drinking beer, waving the national flag and chanting racist slogans.

'Fuck off, Lebs,' they shouted, burning with rage in an attempt to 'reclaim their beach' after a fight between lifesavers and a group of Middle Eastern men. 'We grew here, you flew here,' screamed one group. The TV images and newspaper photographs were confronting: those who looked Middle Eastern were hunted down and beaten.

Broadcast around the globe, the ugly scenes were swiftly condemned as a national disgrace – as 'un-Australian' – and community groups such as Surf Life Saving Australia swung into action, trying to heal the damage through such initiatives as training Muslim swimmers to be lifeguards.

But for Yusra and her family and friends, the damage was deep and long-lasting. For years, her family avoided mainstream beaches like Cronulla and Maroubra, even though they loved them. Instead, they went to quieter, more culturally diverse places, like Sans Souci and Brighton-Le-Sands, on the foreshore of Botany Bay.

'After the riots, there was a palpable fear of going to the other beaches. The riots added to the sense that things really were quite territorial. We all knew that multiculturalism was a wonderful Australian notion' – she smiles sadly, shaking her head – 'but it didn't feel like such diversity extended to the beach.'

Despite the hurt she must feel, there is no trace of rancour as Yusra speaks. She is sitting on the deck of Wylie's Baths, the stately heritage-listed ocean pool in South Coogee, and sipping tea. It's a Friday afternoon and a group of schoolchildren and their mothers troop through the gates, shrieking with excitement. She adjusts her headscarf and continues quietly. 'The images of Middle Easterners being bashed at beaches like Cronulla' – she stops for a moment, then composes herself – 'it repelled us from venturing out of our comfort zone for many years.'

The riots unleashed the same Islamophobia they had experienced after the September 11 attacks in New York, she says. 'There's a pressure placed upon the Muslim community. You almost felt like you were guilty until proved innocent, almost as if you had to be on your best behaviour to prove that you were not a terrorist. Because you know you're dealing with people who have prejudiced views of Muslims – there was a subconscious pressure to show there is nothing to be afraid of.'

The pressure after September 11 was immense, but this time the prejudice was keeping Yusra from one of her great loves, salt water. After the shock of the riots subsided, she decided to fight back. She formed Swim Sisters, a support group for women from all backgrounds to swim regularly and to improve confidence and skills in the open water.

The group of women cut quite a figure as they enter the surf, most clad from crown to ankle in elegant lycra tunics, leggings and matching swim hoods. Heads held high, shoulders pulled back, they approach the turquoise water in their burkinis with confidence and grace.

'Diving into the ocean would have to be one of the most wonderful feelings in the world,' Yusra says. She laughs at the notion that Muslim women can't swim. 'We're all Australians; we're all here to enjoy the ocean. It doesn't matter what you're wearing. It's really important that we have freedom of choice. And besides, once you're in the open water, your choice of swimwear becomes less and less of an issue. We all battle the same waves.' Besides, when the water temperature drops, the burkini blends in with the surrounding wetsuits.

The Swim Sisters became a familiar sight at Bondi once the beaches opened up after COVID-19. With the help of the Bondi Surf Life Saving Club, they took part in a six-week ocean safety program, learning how to understand rips, how to dive under a wave and, eventually, how to catch a wave. Each week, as their confidence grew, Yusra and the Swim Sisters did more and more things in the ocean that they thought they could never do. They swam around the buoys at the back of the bays, about 400–500 metres from shore, and learned how to handle themselves in the surf if they got dumped.

After some weeks, they felt confident enough to start training for 1-kilometre open-water swims. They have since become one of the thrills of Yusra's life. 'I've always loved the ocean, but it's when you're out in the open that it takes on a new dimension. I thought I knew what it felt like to swim, but I didn't really realise what I was missing out on until

~~~

**'After the riots, there was
a palpable fear of going
to the other beaches.'**

~~~

I started swimming out in the open water. It's like discovering another dimension, another world. Especially when you're connecting with marine life.' That's always a buzz, she says, to realise you're among stingrays, or striped or spangled fish, or baby Port Jackson sharks, or even the blue gropers, who come so close she can reach out and touch them. She smiles. 'I can't really put a price on it.'

Yusra has learned to love the unpredictability of the ocean, the way it is a metaphor for life. 'One day it might be as calm as a lake, the next it's rough, and you learn you can't change it, you just have to adapt to it and, if you can, use the conditions to your advantage. You learn to go with the flow. When you're caught in a rip you don't fight it, you just lie on your back. You learn to navigate through the difficulty.'

What has helped the Swim Sisters enormously, she believes, is the warm welcome they have received from Surf Life Saving clubs such as Cronulla, Bronte, Bondi, Coogee and Maroubra. Around a quarter of the people who drown in Australia were born overseas, according to the Royal Life Saving Society – most of whom lacked swimming skills. The need for more ocean swimming skills is therefore great, especially within culturally and linguistically diverse communities. The Swim Sisters have already produced several swimmers strong enough to become surf lifesavers who patrol the beach on weekends.

None of this would be possible without the revolutionary piece of swimwear known as the burkini, designed in 2004 by Lebanese-born, Lakemba-based Aheda Zanetti. Aheda was a stay-at-home mother of three when she designed the garment. Unable to find any sports clothes for her niece, who wore a hijab, she bought a bolt of lycra and carefully cut out and sewed a long tunic and hijood – or swim hood – on her lounge-room floor. Teamed with matching leggings, the burkini was born.

Her niece adored it, and several of her friends asked if Aheda could make one for them too. Word spread. Then, in 2019, model Halima Aden wore a burkini in *Sports Illustrated*, and Aheda's hobby became a global business. A new industry in modesty swimwear was born.

For Yusra, the burkini was nothing short of life-changing, allowing her to pursue her dream of open-water swimming, and embrace Australia's beach culture, while upholding her religious beliefs. Like many Muslim women, she began wearing the hijab as a teenager, as an expression of her faith. Regular Speedos were out of the question, for modesty reasons, at the pool or beach, so she would improvise with long-sleeved T-shirts or rashies, board shorts or leggings. 'I always felt hesitant and shy and timid swimming in public places. There was always this subtle sense of scrutiny and disapproval,' she says. 'I remember people looking at me when I came out of the change rooms as if they were saying, "You're wearing *that*?"'

Swimming carnivals were out of the question.

So she was appalled, as many were, when the Burkini Ban, as it became known, was introduced in various French municipalities in 2016. The ban was based on the grounds that the full-body swimsuit 'conspicuously' shows a person's religion, which goes against French secular principles. In one incident, on a beach in Nice, a French woman dressed in a burkini was approached by police and handed a fine. In footage of the interaction, the woman was shown stripping away her outer garment to bare her neck and arms, under the watchful gaze of all the people surrounding her.

'I found it so alarming to see that women are literally being policed for what they wear,' Yusra says. 'No one has the right to impose their own meaning on a woman's choices. How a woman dresses is her own decision and should not be dictated by men in power.'

Today, she says, the burkini tends to attract admiration and curiosity rather than judgement or fear. 'We often are asked by other women at the beach about where they can buy one. There's a growing club of women who don't want to bare all their flesh in public, or who just want to be more modest.'

Becoming an ocean swimmer has been no easy feat for Yusra, or for her Swim Sisters. For a start, growing up in south-west Sydney meant the shoreline was a 40- to 50-minute drive, often through a snarl of commuter traffic. The ocean remained a mystery to her for a long time: a place of both mesmerising beauty and danger, where the north-east wind brought an armada of bluebottles, with their agonising stings, where sharks could set off the alarms at major beaches, and where rips could carry you far out to sea.

Tides, swells, wind direction and water quality were not part of her everyday conversation, as they often are for those who grow up near the coast. But the ocean called and called to her, as a gravitational pull. She had spent the first nine years of her life in the portside city of Alexandria after all, with her parents, Faten and Wahied, and her siblings. There, the smell and sound of the Mediterranean – its beauty – permeated their lives. They would often walk along the seashore and enjoy meals at outdoor restaurants.

The calm waters of the Mediterranean are a world away from Sydney's wild and unpredictable surf beaches, though. The bays and beaches of Alexandria were something to gently dip in and out of rather than race across in a swim squad, often in big waves. So, once they had settled in Sydney, Faten and Wahied enrolled Yusra and her three siblings in classes at Greenacre Swimming Centre, a classic 25-metre suburban pool not far from their home.

The pool was a social hub for the local Arabic-speaking community. On sweltering days mothers in hijabs would congregate under the shade of the gum trees to share food and gossip as their toddlers ran across the lawn. Youngsters splashed in shallow pools under the eagle eyes of their parents. It was there that Yusra learned to dog paddle up and down the pool, loving the cool embrace of it, how it made her feel weightless and free. Later, the burkini gave her the confidence to take adult swimming classes, where she learned freestyle, and then, finally, to plunge into the ocean with the Swim Sisters.

These days – with a toddler often underfoot, and part-time work as a solicitor – her aim when she swims is not so much to compete in ocean marathons but to clear her head, and to feel strong. She loves the sense of freedom, the calm and serenity that settle over her after being immersed in salt water.

'Swimming itself is a sort of meditation, or a way of cultivating a sense of wonder, or being at one with nature. I feel mesmerised by the beauty of all the things God creates when I'm in the water,' she says. 'You're alone in his creation – you're with the fish, and the coral and the seaweed. I feel a strong connection to the Creator whenever I'm swimming.'

There is a strong parallel, in fact, between swimming with a group and praying in her mosque. 'On one hand you're in a group, but then when you're head down, you are ultimately alone in the water, as you are in prayer.'

Lately, Yusra has been taking herself to McIver's Ladies Baths, a Victorian treasure at Coogee Beach. A curtain of peace descends as you walk down the steps into the baths. You pay an entry fee of $2.50 at the quaint clubhouse, which was deliberately set on fire in the 1980s by someone unable to accept that this was strictly a women's and children's only space. A little further down – past the outdoor shower and the change rooms overlooking Wedding Cake Island and the Pacific – are women of all shapes and sizes, from every faith and every country, basking on the warm rock ledges, doing breaststroke or just floating in the body of turquoise water cut into the sandstone.

McIver's had been healing women for a long time; legend has it that it was a bathing and birthing place for Bidjigal and Gadigal women. It's still the place many women naturally gravitate to when they are pregnant, or wanting to bring their babies to the ocean for the first time. Or when they want to swim a few peaceful laps without anyone tailgating them, or they're recovering from surgery or simply want to rest and heal, away from the pressure of the public gaze.

Yusra first discovered the solace of this place as a nineteen-year-old, and then reconnected to the pool when she fell pregnant five years ago. With swollen limbs and feet, she found it soothing and freeing to stretch out in the salt water. As she neared the end of her pregnancy she would visit in the late afternoon, after her antenatal appointments, and sometimes felt the unexpected joy of having this special body of water all to herself. She was swimming there just hours before she went into labour with her first child, who is now four years old. 'I was thinking of all the women who had come before me and the fact that it was considered a

'When I'm sitting here at the Ladies Baths, I feel a sense of the universality of the human experience.'

sacred space for Aboriginal women. I'm sure it put me into the right headspace.'

Recently she has been visiting to process the trauma of the scenes unfolding in the Middle East, letting her tears flow freely as she sits on the lawn and gazes out across the ocean. 'Because the news is streaming from our phones now rather than just the filtered TV news, it feels much closer and relatable. It's so graphic and distressing. You see the faces of people who could be your family as their homes and their cities are obliterated by an air strike. You see mothers wailing and weeping over their dead babies, you see a man digging helplessly through the rubble, calling out for his children. You see a child shaking uncontrollably because his home has just collapsed behind him in a bomb blast.'

As the last rays of sunshine touch the pool, Yusra grows thoughtful. 'There are faces you can't get out of your mind. Innocent children who are the ages of my son, nieces and nephews. I have felt worn down but I also know it's important not to look away. You can't ignore human suffering and loss of life.

'Looking across the horizon makes me feel a great sense of solidarity with the women and children in the Middle East … that it is just on the other side of the ocean. When I'm sitting here at the Ladies Baths, I feel a sense of the universality of the human experience. It's a hidden sanctuary for me.'

Where she feels closest to God, she says, is after a swim at Wylie's Baths. Recently she settled her towel in a secluded nook under the large timber deck beside the pool, and used it as a prayer mat. She gazed down at the compass needle on her phone app, which spun, pointing her in the direction of Mecca. She kneeled down and bowed four times before reciting her prayers from the Qur'an. They help her 'detach from worldly concerns and connect to Allah'.

'We have a tradition in our faith of what's called ablution, or ritual purification, whereby you cleanse yourself with water – you wash your mouth, your nose, your feet, the top of your head.' She gestures to each, as she explains. 'To me, ocean swimming doubles as a way to purify oneself, getting me ready to perform my prayer. Even the act of entering is a part of the prayer process – you are washing away your sorrows. Swimming here is incredibly healing.'

Recently, Yusra has returned to Cronulla Beach – first for a family barbecue, with her toddler, and then, later, for a swim on her own. She was understandably apprehensive. 'Never in a million years would I have thought I'd come and change into my burkini in a public toilet – in Cronulla, on my own,' she says. 'I didn't step foot here for almost ten years after the Cronulla riots.'

But as she walked towards the change rooms she noticed a large sticker under the female sign on the toilets. It read: *Show love not fear*. As she dived in and headed out into deep water, she felt the sense of freedom and release that only comes from immersion in salt water. It had been a long wait, but Yusra finally felt at home again in the sea around her.

CHAPTER 8

TIM WINTON

Saving Ningaloo

~~~~

AS WELL AS being something to respect, and to reckon with, the sea has always reassured Australian author Tim Winton. At lunchtime in his Perth primary school, Tim's boyish anxieties were soothed by the sight of the bombora – the large sea waves breaking out over a submerged reef. His family may have lived 5 kilometres inland, in a house with no view of the ocean, but in the afternoons, as he buckled down to his homework, the cool sea breeze known as the Fremantle Doctor would arrive, lifting his spirits as it rustled the treetops and stirred the curtains.

Christmas holidays heralded their annual migration, for six weeks, to his family's holiday shack south of Geraldton, where the surf 'hammered night and day'. Most days, he would wake before dawn to go crayfishing with his father. He savoured every moment of those days, either in, on or beside the salt water.

But it was when Tim was twelve, and his father's job required his family to suddenly move to Albany, 400 kilometres south of Perth, that the enchantment truly took hold. Feeling 'dislocated, lonely, scared, isolated', he was consoled by the empty white beaches of the West Australian coast. At Cheynes Beach, Waychinicup and Cape Riche, he fished, surfed, foraged and climbed granite headlands with friends. They had, he says, 'a hell of a time', camping, diving for abalone and cooking on open fires.

'I found solace in the place long before I found it in any social setting,' he says. 'In this regard I'm probably not so different now. While I get to choose where I live these days, I still need places as much as people. I think nature and exercise have antidepressant effects – that's a pretty safe scientific view now – and adolescence is a time of turmoil and confusion. (So is middle age, for that matter.) Nature brings me back to people in better shape. That's good for me, and probably good for the people in my life.'

He found the ocean, in particular, a 'very rich sensory environment. All that movement, all those smells, all that effervescence.' Despite the fact that he came from a loving,

132

supportive family, he burned with angst when adolescent hormones kicked in. 'I was frustrated, impatient, confused, angry. I think it was enormously liberating. To be alone with the sea – that was great. I felt mastered by the sea. Held. I always got out of the water feeling better than when I got in. I often say it was like a huge salty poultice sucking the poison out of me, and I think that's how it remains for me all these years later.'

Freediving was therapeutic too. In *Land's Edge*, Tim's much-loved homage to the Western Australian coast, he describes diving as 'like gliding, flying, the country unfolding below'. He began descending deeper into the water, and for longer, to the point where 'the pressure rings the changes through my whole body'.

'These moments in extremis can be revelatory as well as painful or uncomfortable (or just bloody scary),' he says. 'It's like fasting. Your senses are sharpened. You're receptive in ways you may not be when you're more sedentary or comfortable. Water makes you nearly weightless. Gravity is our gift and burden. To be free of it for a while can be a blessing.'

It seems only natural, then, that this love affair with the coast would coruscate through his books. *Cloudstreet*, *Breath* and *Dirt Music* thrum with the boom of Indian Ocean breakers, and *Land's Edge* and *Island Home* have helped stamp the beauty and the terrors of the Australian coast deep into our psyches.

And, as Tim was immortalising our coastline in writing, it began to change him too. Little would he have known, spearfishing along the coast in his youth, that he would one day become an environmental activist who would, among other things, be instrumental in saving Ningaloo Reef, 'one of the last wild places in the world'.

The world's largest fringing coral reef, 1200 kilometres north of Perth, Ningaloo is a wonderland of coral, brimming with dugongs, turtles, sharks and stingrays. From a boat you can swim with the largest fish in the world, the 8-metre whale shark. You might, if you're lucky, spot a humpback whale looking after its calf in the sheltered waters of Exmouth Gulf, known as 'Ningaloo's nursery'. Tim loves the place fiercely; he has swum, dived, snorkelled and walked along every part of it, and now defends it 'like kin'.

The transformation began slowly enough, almost by osmosis, as he began encountering 'large, sometimes rare and endangered marine creatures – turtles, dugongs, manta rays and so on'. 'Being up close and personal to so many unique marine animals is instructive,' he says. They changed the way he saw the world. 'We share this planet with other species, and everything is connected and interdependent.'

His 'peak' experience, he says, was 'being face to face with a curious humpback whale and her calf. A massive, intelligent animal right up in your grille for twenty minutes – something that could crush you like a bug at any moment and yet wants to check you out very carefully at slightly terrifying

'Nature brings me back
to people in better shape.
That's good for me, and
probably good for the
people in my life.'

proximity – that's up there. There's something special about being up close to an animal that big.

'I've had animals that become familiar, like blue gropers. I think a lot of folks have experienced very benign and uplifting moments with gropers and big cods, encounters that allow them to feel closer to another wild species than they'd normally be able to get. Aside from the thrill and the emotional uplift, I think these are instructive encounters. Many of us live a kind of denatured existence that impoverishes us and puts the health of the natural world at risk at the same time.'

Part of getting to know marine life entailed appreciating its possibilities. Cetaceans, for instance – whales, dolphins and porpoises – 'are smart and curious ... and show moments of altruism' but, he acknowledges, 'they can also be unbelievably brutal'. So can the sea itself. Despite the saying that 'you never regret a swim', Tim has had moments when he's felt as if the ocean was pushing him away. He particularly detests stingers. 'I can take a few pings and dings on a swim, but copping a flogging is no fun. Also, sometimes you just make the wrong call and wind up on your arse on an oyster reef getting cut to ribbons. But that's just operator error. Know your water. Know your limits.'

More than once he has almost drowned. 'It's not an experience I'd recommend,' he says. The first time was when he was nine years old, and his boat capsized on a reef. What that taught him was that the ocean 'is bigger than me and it doesn't give a damn'. He has remained in awe of its power ever since. 'I've saved a few folks (mostly kids) from drowning over the years. It happens so quickly, this transition from being safe to being in death's mouth. You're a small creature in the scheme of things, and although your ancestral home is the sea, you're only a semi-skilled citizen in that medium. Everything is contingent. No matter how literate you are in ocean stuff, no matter how skilled you've become, conditions change quickly.'

It was *Blueback*, the children's story he wrote in 1997, that set him on the path towards ocean stewardship. Its protagonists, Abel Jackson and his mother, Dora, battle to save the ocean near their home from developers. He wrote *Blueback* in a week, oblivious to the fact that Dora would hold him to account for the rest of his life, and that the book would inspire many readers – as well as Tim himself – to become activists.

Dora, like Tim, finds inspiration in the seminal book *The Sea Around Us*, by the late marine biologist Rachel Carson. Carson called the ocean 'the great mother of life'. Tim agrees. 'Our fate is inextricably linked to the fortunes of the sea: when it dies, so do we,' he writes. As she contemplates the damage that the developers would do to the ocean, Dora reaches the same conclusion. 'We come from water,' she says. 'We belong to it.'

'Our fate is inextricably
linked to the fortunes of the
sea: when it dies, so do we.'

The sea, in this way, has value beyond what many ascribe to it. Tim is aware of this – almost painfully, at times – and for years has understood that certain parts of our oceans have a particularly powerful – almost sacred – presence. 'This isn't always just to do with their physical grandeur, which Westerners are most susceptible to. Sometimes they're places of increase – fertility, nurture, abundance. Nursery environments are particularly notable in this regard. Lagoons and shorelines where, for thousands of years, turtles have come back to mate and nest. Mangroves and seagrass meadows where dugongs aggregate. Calm bays where whales give birth and nurse their calves. These aren't just important places for the species involved. For millennia they've been crucial to humans as well. Animals and humans inscribe themselves onto places, but it's worth remembering that places inscribe themselves onto humans and animals too.'

So when, in 2000, a developer tried to build a luxury marina resort on the shores of Ningaloo Reef, which would have swelled the population to thousands and introduced hundreds of powerboats, causing more pollution and overdevelopment, Tim became the public face of the campaign to save it. 'Getting government and commerce to pull up – that requires serious work,' he says. Thankfully, many activists joined him. With his imprimatur, and the power of tens of thousands of people marching, protesting, writing letters and holding endless meetings, government policy was changed and Ningaloo was spared. It was later put on the World Heritage list.

The experience gave him great faith in people power. 'Here was this remote, obscure place that thousands of ordinary folks decided to fight for, despite never having been there. It was the variety of people across generations, class boundaries and political affiliations that told me something was up, something different was going on,' he says.

And it wasn't hopeless. In his lifetime, Tim has seen whales brought back from the brink of extinction. As a teenager in Albany, on Western Australia's South Coast, he'd watched sperm whales being hoisted up onto flensing decks and hacked up by men in beanies for cosmetics and fertiliser. It was visceral. 'Tourists could go out to the whaling station and watch them being chopped up. It was a pretty ghastly thing to witness,' he recalls. 'It stank like nothing you've ever smelled in your life.

'What was most offensive was knowing that the industry understood how close to extinction sperm and humpback whales were by then, and yet they were determined to press on with business as usual. That was where I learned that business can deploy apparently rational language in the pursuit of utterly irrational activities. Conservationists quoted the science as a reason to stop whaling, but industry said the greenies were emotive and hysterical and so did the media. Which sounds pretty familiar from today's experience with the climate crisis, right? When whaling finally ended here in 1978, there were 300 humpbacks left in the western population and now there are probably 40,000. It shows what we can achieve if we wake up and pull up before it's too late.'

Ningaloo was declared a World Heritage Site in 2011 and, since then, Tim has continued to steadfastly defend it in the hope that the nearby, and equally important, Exmouth Gulf – which is a nursery for humpback whales, dugongs and critically endangered sawfish – will also garner World Heritage protection. He recently wrote, narrated and produced the three-part ABC series *Ningaloo Nyinggulu*, to raise awareness of the importance of supporting various ecosystems. It shows him immersed in turquoise waters, helping scientists to hold a 450-kilogram dugong to tag and track it, as well as diving with whale sharks to help pick parasites off their gums. He describes the process as like 'hanging off the front of a bus'. When he returns to the boat at this point in the documentary, he is almost speechless with amazement.

Tim first swam with whale sharks in his thirties. He found the 8-metre fish – with a tail that 'swings like a factory gate' – intimidating in its size but also saw such experiences as 'inspiring, almost religious in their nature'. Thirty years later, in the filming of the documentary, and despite the water around him being 'full of camera folks jostling to get the shots', it still felt like a 'real privilege' to swim with such a giant animal. 'Given how rare it is to be allowed to touch megafauna, that was a great moment.'

There's only one shot in the documentary of the greatest threat to Ningaloo: the fossil fuel industry. At the end,

Chevron's massive Wheatstone gas facility, near Onslow, comes into view. This was deliberate. 'We wanted to focus on the glories of Ningaloo, to show what's there, what we have to celebrate – thanks to good luck and the hard work of conservationists – but also what we have to lose if we don't wake up,' he says.

And besides, 'the visual imagery of oil and gas operations never really does justice to the sensory experience of being close to them'. You can imagine him scowling as he says this. 'The smells, the roaring noise, the hellish night-time daylight for kilometres all around, the sinister vibration, the uncanny feeling of being in the presence of something ingenious and monstrous that's supposed to be civil but actually feels military. Some oil and gas companies have assets and influence larger than nation states, including armies. It's hard to convey all that in a few seconds, or even minutes, in a visual medium. It needs its own doco.'

Tim feels indebted to Ningaloo not only for the inspiration it has given him as a writer but also for what it has taught him about the importance of the wild. 'I think Ningaloo provided me with an education beyond anything the academy had afforded me. Not just in matters of marine science, either. I mean across the board, in every aspect of life. It helped me appreciate how precious life is. We're a species evolved from wild places. Wild places are our nursery and lifeblood. Functioning ecosystems are the foundation of all life, human life included, and for quite a while now we've trained ourselves to think of ourselves as existing outside of nature, of mastering nature to the point of superseding it. This isn't just hubris, it's folly. In the short term, it's making us miserable. Eventually it'll render us hungry and then homeless. Wild places are a measure of our health and our future. They're also points of reconnection and perspective.'

What Tim found humbling, in making the documentary, was realising that his connection to the place is fleeting compared to that of the First Peoples of Ningaloo, the Baiyungu people, whose footsteps go back more than 60,000 years. The reef's traditional custodians played a critical role in the making of the program; it was 'deeply moving', Tim says, to sit next to Baiyungu Elder Hazel Walgar on the floor of a rock shelter, overlooking the ocean, as she paid homage to her ancestral home.

'There were people in Ningaloo when there were Neanderthals in Europe,' he says. They were 'forced off their ancestral lands by invasion and colonisation. Settlers, pastoralists, police and governments abused them, starved them, imprisoned them, murdered them and sent them into miserable exile.'

Even worse, they were told they never existed. The Baiyungu people only received native title in 2019. 'I've known Hazel for a while,' Tim says, 'and I know a little bit about what her family's been through. We're of the same generation and yet we've lived very different lives. It's pretty awe-inspiring to sit in the dirt, surrounded by ancient artefacts, but to be there with someone whose ancestors made and used those tools and made the cooking fires and ate the foods associated with those bones and shells, that was special.'

In one sequence in the series, Hazel talks about the Mandu Mandu beads, the oldest symbolic ornament on the continent, to which she and her family are linked and which her relatives helped archaeologists uncover in the 1980s. 'Hazel's older sister Gwen was at the first public screening [of the documentary],' Tim recalls, 'and her response to what was happening on-screen during those moments was visceral. After so much loss and longing and sorrow, moments of return and vindication like that are massive.

'Few of us raised in comfort and security can understand how important these moments of recognition and return are. It was a window into another existence, an opportunity that's so often offered to non-Indigenous Australians but one that's mostly spurned. Aboriginal Australians are, in my experience, enormously forbearing and generous. It's shameful how easily this forbearance and generosity can be taken for granted or dismissed by mainstream folks. This ignorance and contempt hurts all of us, impoverishes all of us, distorts and stunts all of us.'

First Nations People have vital information to share with the wider culture, including government, about how to look after our oceans. They have been talking about two-way thinking for generations now, Tim says. By this, he is referring to a desire to share the knowledge they have absorbed from living continuously in the natural world for tens of thousands of years, and for that sharing and respect to be reciprocated.

Our science, arts and social policies will only benefit if we listen, he says. 'Aboriginal people have 60,000 years of experience and expertise to deploy and to offer the rest of the culture, and we ignore this at our peril. I know senior scientists in several fields who've copped to this in recent years and who say they wished they'd woken up to it decades ago. The future of our oceans – indeed our planet – depends on deeper knowledge married to an ethic of restraint. The science community has come to realise this. Indigenous stewards have always known this.'

Meanwhile, climate change remains foremost in Tim's mind. 'None of our efforts will mean a thing if we have a disordered and dangerous climate. The science has made it plain. We have to stop new fossil-fuel developments and wind down our use of oil and gas quickly. Citizens who want to defend their children's and grandchildren's futures need to demand that this happens. Fossil-fuel businesses are already on the nose. They're making billions. Many, like Woodside and Chevron and Santos, don't want to change. Quite a few of them are working to undermine any positive change. But people have come to see through that. They see those politicians who are essentially doing their bidding. But business as usual is beginning to unravel. Ordinary folks have ways to accelerate that process by not investing in these companies, not banking with financial institutions that fund them, calling for all forms of state capture and dirty sponsorship to cease.'

There are many specific, tangible things we can do, he says. Vote for representatives who are serious about climate. Boycott businesses that put our grandchildren's futures in jeopardy. Join others to get organised and raise a common voice. 'That's how we've achieved every significant bit of social and policy progress in this country. It's okay to be concerned. It's sensible to be angry. But none of us can do this on our own. We'll need each other if we want to save the seas and the planet from business as usual.'

Soberingly, he says, since saving Ningaloo, 'things have gotten far worse and declined at a rate even worse than expected. I live most of the year now in a region that's quickly becoming uninsurable because of global heating. That's something being experienced right now on both sides of the continent in the north. On current trends, with current policy settings, I don't think my grandchildren are likely to be able to live there as adults. Their kids may not even be able to visit at all. In the past few years, I've seen coral reefs bleach where bleaching is rare. So, yes, climate change is front of mind now, not an exception, and not a distant looming prospect. It's upon us and we're flailing.'

One of the most shocking signals of human impact on the ocean came in 2011, when Tim witnessed thousands of abalone stranded on the beach. There had been a marine heatwave, and, because they'd found the water too hot, the abalone had sought out cooler climes. The searing beach, unfortunately, could not provide relief. His concern for the environment suddenly took on a new level of urgency.

~~~

'Climate change is front of mind now and not a distant looming prospect. It's upon us and we're flailing.'

~~~

'Well, we're all in that slow-boiling frog scenario, aren't we?' he says. 'But now and then you really feel the heat and react. That heatwave was momentous and horrible, and abalone is a big part of my family culture. I'm not sure if I'll ever be able to gather abalone again on the mid-west coast, where I grew up diving for it.'

There are dark days when Tim despairs about opportunities squandered when it comes to marine conservation, particularly the efforts that went into establishing marine parks around the country. Forty-two marine reserves, covering more than 100,000 square kilometres, were set up as protected zones in 2012, which was a great achievement, Tim says. But it didn't last; the plan was suspended a year later, in a move that conservationists regarded as a huge step backwards. 'When Tony Abbott got elected shortly thereafter, that once-in-a-lifetime achievement was butchered. Similarly, the Sydney Marine Park was a great achievement betrayed by cowardice.'

So what gives him hope? The next generation. 'Young people understand what the old suits are doing. They're fed up with being robbed and lied to. Change is coming, be assured (or terrified) of that.'

He also remains encouraged by the gradual shift in the appreciation of, and respect for, the fragility of our marine ecology. Lately, this has involved 'seeing the sorrow and outrage people are showing every time some knucklehead spears a blue groper that's known and loved by a local community. That shows you things have changed. A few years ago, a bloke holding up a 25-year-old fish on a spear was a hero. Now he's a bit of a tool. When I was a boy, Ron and Val Taylor were shark killers. Now Val's a conservation ambassador. That's an arc of progress right there.'

Tim is too unassuming to claim that his activism has threatened his livelihood or his family. What he will admit, though, is that 'every action, every human value, comes at a cost. And we have learned to be careful.'

At 63, Tim follows the same rhythm he did as a boy: the mornings are for being outdoors – fishing, swimming, diving, beachcombing, with the same sense of 'humility and awe'. The afternoons are for writing and reading. He lives in a fibro house with sand dunes at his back door in a small 'redneck' crayfishing town on the west coast. It's a place of 'merciless weather, a flat and barren affair'. Almost every day, he goes to the sea. And, just as it did when he was a boy, it reassures him. On the days he can't get there, the smell of 'rotting sea grass and the blast of the Fremantle Doctor' remind him it's close.

Whenever he goes abroad, the first thing he does when he comes home is to stand on the beach looking westwards, with the continent behind him. Because this is, after all, his island home, and there is nowhere else in the world he would rather be.

CHAPTER 9

ERIKA GLEESON AND DIPPERS

Swimming Upstream

~~~

SYDNEY'S BRONTE BEACH is a mere 250 metres wide, but what it lacks in size it makes up for in an abundance of what the late artist Brett Whiteley called 'optical ecstasy'. Its bottle-green breakers – which can be wild and dangerous – are wedged between two sandstone cliffs in Sydney's Eastern Suburbs, studded with multimillion-dollar homes. To one side are the Bronte Baths, built in 1887, and behind it lies a verdant swathe of bushland filled with paperbarks, she-oaks and wattles.

It is a progressive as well as a startlingly beautiful place. You'd have to have a heart of stone not to feel uplifted by the new surf education program the Bronte Surf Life Saving Club has recently embraced. On Saturday mornings over the summer months, the participants of the Dippers program – many of whom are neurodivergent and often terrified of the beach – are gradually encouraged, week by week, year by year, to put their toes in the sand or dip their hands at the water's edge. With equal doses of patience and encouragement, they may learn to relax enough to put their face in the water for a few moments.

For Moorebank mum Chloe Alder, taking her two sons, Harley and Jasper, to Dippers has been life-changing. Chloe first noticed Harley was different when he was a toddler. 'He would obsessively open and shut the glass doors onto our apartment balcony. When I'd ask him to stop, he would have a complete meltdown,' she recalls. 'At one point we had a box made especially for him with a glass door so he could open and close it as much as he liked.'

Harley's speech was quirky. Instead of asking for a drink, he would repeatedly mimic his mother, asking her in a sing-song, high-pitched voice, 'Do you want a drink, Harley?' He had an uncanny flair for letters and numbers and shapes. 'He could see patterns in numbers, and knew the alphabet when he was fifteen months.'

Chloe felt 'blindsided' the day a paediatrician gave her the diagnosis that Harley was on the autism spectrum.

'You worry about everything. How is he going to cope in life? Who is going to look after him when I'm not here? Is anyone going to take advantage of him? He's going to face so many challenges in life. And there is a stigma associated with autism,' she says. 'I knew it was a long, rocky road ahead.'

Her second son, Jasper, also struggled in group settings, and floundered when it came to listening and following directions. The diagnosis that he too was on the autism spectrum made her doubly determined to find as much help as she could for her sons. Speech therapy, occupational therapy and group therapy followed in quick succession. She took the boys to see a GP, a paediatrician and a family therapist. She joined a carers group and a disability playgroup. She took both her sons to classes at the local swimming school but, like a lot of children with a disability, they were unable to filter out the raucous sounds around them and concentrate on the teacher's instructions. They'd end up having a tantrum or getting into an argument with others.

'You desperately want them to have the same opportunities as everyone else,' she says. 'I was at my wit's end, wondering what could help them.' When she found out about Dippers, she signed up in a heartbeat.

At first Harley was daunted by the group sessions at Coogee Beach. 'He gets sensory overload easily, and finds free time difficult,' Chloe says. 'He likes structure and routine.' But each Saturday morning, a Dippers volunteer would patiently spend hours by Harley's side as he explored the wooden fishing boats that had been pulled up onto the sand at the north end of the beach. He would walk around with a stuffed toy, fascinated by the signposts saying *Swim Between the Flags* or *Dangerous Rip*. His favourite place on the beach was the giant rainbow painted on the semicircular steps leading down to the sand; he would lie down on it every week, grinning madly.

There was never any pressure for Harley to take part in any of the activities, or any rush to succeed. Slowly, week by week, he grew accustomed to the sound of the waves, and the seagulls, and the sounds of other people, and began enjoying himself on the sand and in the water. He now regards Dippers as his favourite thing in the world. Ask him about his Saturday mornings with the group and it's like turning on a tap. 'Dippers,' he says, beaming, 'is totally awesome. I wish it happened all the time.'

So how did he feel when he first began? 'Beach-cited,' he says. 'I was worried I would sink in the water,' he explains. 'All I wanted to do was run away. But I don't do that anymore.' Now, he says, when he goes to the ocean baths, he likes looking for shells, fish and crabs; when he's really lucky, he might find a coin. 'We also do hurdles and make sandcastles. I wish we could make water castles, but that doesn't work.'

The first time he jumped in the water is tattooed in his mind. 'Oh, we jumped over waves, I remember that! And there was a big frog floaty thing there.' (A flotation device called a lily pad.) One Saturday morning, with the volunteers

~~~

Chloe felt 'blindsided' the day a paediatrician gave her the diagnosis that Harley was on the autism spectrum. 'You worry about everything. How is he going to cope in life?'

~~~

helping him, Harley scrambled up onto a boogie board and rode a small wave back to shore. 'I just couldn't believe that was him,' Chloe recalls. 'I seriously never thought I would see him do something like that.'

The benefits have flowed through to the rest of Harley's life. 'When he's out near the water now, that's the most content and at peace he ever is. And those few hours after we come home would have to be the happiest few hours we have all week. Getting in the water just seemed to have such a powerful effect on him. He's become a much happier person, much more confident with people,' she says. 'He actually makes eye contact with people or smiles at them.'

It wasn't long before Dippers was working its magic on Chloe's second son. Jasper's needs were very different to his older brother's. 'He was just champing at the bit to get in the water. If we didn't hold him back, he would have jumped in and started heading to New Zealand.'

Born with low muscle tone, Jasper tires quickly, and needed to build his fitness as well as learning the ins and outs of water safety skills. 'He tended to become exhausted when he was on the shore with the waves crashing around him,' Chloe says. 'Then he'd panic. But the Dippers team slowly taught him to calm down, build up his strength, and become more confident in the water.'

Jasper admits that, like his brother, he was slow to warm to the program. 'But now I'm really good at it,' he says. 'I learned how to go under the waves by holding my breath and closing my eyes. I learned that you stay between the flags – I think because between the flags is the best water. I also learned how to get to the lily pad to jump off, which was really cool.'

The miracle worker behind Dippers is Erika Gleeson, a 35-year-old behaviour specialist working with those who are on the autism spectrum or have an intellectual disability. She grew up in the small coastal northern NSW town of Port Macquarie, and spent her childhood riding bodyboards in the whitewash with her friends.

When she began supporting people with disabilities, she was hooked. Her eyes glint like the sea when she talks about her work. 'I knew this was something I wanted to do for the rest of my life. I find people I work with more fascinating than neurotypicals. I definitely don't see them as "inspirational".' She frowns at that idea. 'I just love identifying where they need some additional support in order for them to reach their potential.'

Erika realised how beneficial swimming was for her clients when she noticed one of them, a teenager named Paddy who was on the autism spectrum, transform into a 'different kid' whenever he got into the local pool. 'It was just incredible. He was so happy, so absorbed in his world, he didn't listen to a word I was saying. I learned to just let him relax and

The pressure of the water around them is ... almost like being held, like a hug. It calms down their nervous system.

have fun, while keeping an eagle eye on him, and then slowly working towards some goals.'

Erika pauses to watch a ferry leave Circular Quay and plough its way across the emerald water of Sydney Harbour. 'Why shouldn't everyone be able to enjoy the ocean and the beach?' She was shocked to discover, during these first few years in the disability sector, that 90 per cent of deaths of autistic children are the result of drowning. 'Their need for water skills was actually far greater than most.' To her dismay, though, the swim schools and surf clubs she approached seemed unwilling or unable to include people with diverse needs into their classes. So Erika took matters into her own hands. She set up a training course for aquatic professionals called Autism Swim, to give them the knowledge, skills and resources to help people of all ages and abilities.

Soon after, she set up her first Dippers group, run in conjunction with Coogee Surf Life Saving Club. Unlike the Nippers program, which teaches children basic lifesaving techniques, to swim in the open water for hundreds of metres and to race on boards, Dippers has much simpler, but equally important, goals. Some of its students are on the autism spectrum, others have Down syndrome; some have epilepsy, an intellectual disability or visual or hearing impairments. Sometimes they have a combination of these conditions. Often they struggle in supermarkets, school or the workplace. They are prone to panic or being overwhelmed in the cacophony of public swimming pools. 'The water should be for everyone, no matter what their needs, goals and preferences,' Erika says. 'Everyone has the ability to swim and surf with the requisite support. People with disabilities should be able to do what everyone else can do. It's about society becoming more inclusive and more adaptive to everyone's needs.'

The parents of Erika's first group noticed that their children seemed to make huge headway in a relatively short amount of time. Word spread quickly; within a few years, her program had been adopted by progressive surf clubs such as Bronte, Coogee, Bondi, Port Macquarie, Warriewood and Coolangatta.

The backbone of the Dippers program is its volunteers, who are trained to vary the routine to suit the participants' needs and goals. Often the youngsters have trouble communicating or concentrating, or are unsettled by a change in routine. Some don't like loud sounds. Others don't like to be touched. Some have delayed learning and are highly anxious. Some, with no sense of risk, want to paddle out towards the horizon on a boogie board and need to be watched like a hawk.

To communicate with their young charges, especially those who are non-verbal, the volunteers sometimes use visual storyboards, showing the activities of the day – tug of war, relays, board riding. Peter Daly, who has been volunteering at Bronte since the program began, says it's enormously fulfilling to build a rapport with the kids, and watch them grow in confidence as the summer unfolds.

'We get as much out of the program as the parents and families themselves.'

As always, the healing powers of the ocean are at work. Volunteer and occupational therapist Ashleigh Ehrenfeld says she's noticed how immersion in salt water has a deeply therapeutic effect for children with a disability. 'The pressure of the water around them is calming – it's almost like being held, like a hug. It calms down their nervous system. Then add the salt water – whatever the mysterious quality of it is, perhaps the minerals – and on top of that, the soothing sound of the waves, and it seems to do nothing short of working miracles.'

One recent Saturday morning, after gazing at it longingly for years, Harley finally plucked up the courage to go for a ride on one of Coogee Surf Life Saving Club's inflatable rescue boats. After securing him, the lifesavers zoomed about at the back of the beach. Harley is almost lost for words as he tries to describe the euphoria of bouncing and skimming over the glittering waves that day. It seems to be on par with the excitement of landing on the moon. 'I went into the deep, deep water so I swim and go on the boat,' he says. 'That was awesome!'

He was euphoric for hours when he returned, covered in sea spray. 'He simply could not stop talking about it,' Chloe remembers. 'He says going out on the boat is the best thing he's ever done in his life. He is so proud of that moment.'

CHAPTER 10

RAJBIR KAUR
AND
SUMIT SINGH

Little Fish

~~~

PREP WORK FOR dinner is usually well underway by the time Sumit Singh arrives at the GurTaj Indian Restaurant in Collaroy on Sydney's Northern Beaches. It is a noisy business. By 11.30 am his sister-in-law is head down in the kitchen, deep-frying pappadums in vats of vegetable oil. Next to her, another cook is clanging a large frying pan, mixing garam masala, cumin, coriander, turmeric and chilli into a sauce for chicken tikka curry.

With the glass doors flung open, the restaurant is filled with the sound of commuter buses rumbling along Pittwater

Road and talkback radio from a nearby building site. The phone is ringing for reservations, and Sumit's four-year-old son Kuwar is watching *Bluey* on his iPad and banging his teaspoon on the table as he wolfs down a bowl of ice cream.

Sumit exudes a calm, quiet focus amid the rush and din of the family business. Sporting a turban and long beard, he brings a jug of water and a glass to the table, and orders plates of clay oven–baked naan bread, basmati rice and vegetable curry before taking a seat.

What helps him keep a clear mind – and exuberant health – is swimming as often as he can at Freshwater Rockpool, the 50-metre ocean pool tucked under the cliff at the northern end of Freshwater Beach. It takes Sumit ten minutes to drive there, but it makes an enormous difference to the quality of his day.

As he walks towards it, he leaves behind the incessant pings of his phone, email and other technological sounds. When he slides into the pool, he is enveloped by the sounds of nature: waves crashing on the shore and the rocks, the languid strokes of other swimmers, the wind in the trees, birds singing and the sound of his own breath. As his arms pull him through the glinting water, his mood is transformed. He doesn't know exactly how it happens but, as his breath slows and he glides from one end of the pool to the other, there is a shift in his perception.

'Running a restaurant means you are always looking for a solution to things,' he says, nodding to his wife, Raaj, as she arrives to help set up the front of house. 'Something always

~~~

As his breath slows and he glides from one end of the pool to the other, there is a shift in his perception.

~~~

happens by the third lap – I've often worked out how to fix a problem I've been mulling over.'

He swims right through winter, wearing only board shorts. His one concession to the cold – and hypothermia – is putting the heater on full blast in his car before and after his swim. He also wears a swim cap with extra room for his long, thick hair. Over that, he pulls on a 5-millimetre-thick neoprene swim cap that covers his ears and keeps his head warm.

The long hair and turban are important to his Sikh faith, he says, a symbol of their devotion to God. 'If you are travelling in India, and you're in trouble – say you've missed your bus and it's dark or you've lost your wallet and need to get home, all you have to do is stand next to someone in a turban. Their job is to help you out.'

When he returns to work after swimming in the salt water – especially cold salt water – it is with a sense of accomplishment. 'The first quarter of the lap can be a bit painful in winter,' he says. 'But it's best not to think about it too much. I just get in and start swimming. It makes me incredibly efficient when I get back to work. I always make the hardest phone calls as soon as I get out of the pool, sitting in the car, or on the way back. That's when I am my most grounded.'

But there is another, deeper benefit that flows from his swim: the feel-good factor of mastering a skill that had long eluded him. Like many other migrants, Sumit learned to swim as an adult. He was twelve when he and his parents arrived in Sydney from Punjab, a productive, prosperous state in north-west India. Sumit's father, Gusharan, was a code breaker in the Indian army before he decided to migrate to Sydney in his thirties, hoping for a better future for his family. Unable to find equivalent work here, he rolled his sleeves up and learned to cook at his cousin's restaurant in Crows Nest. He had little money and few connections, but he worked hard and saved hard and, in 1996, he opened up a small takeaway serving curries near Collaroy Beach. The locals loved it, and when he moved to a larger restaurant nearby, they followed.

Gusharan is 70 now and sits on the back wall of the restaurant, a great glowing mountain of a man who meticulously checks the pots as the chefs bring them out from the kitchen for him to taste. He thumps his chest. 'My cooking comes from my heart. That's just as important as skills in the kitchen.'

Punjab is a landlocked state, and swimming was not a skill many of its people put much thought into. Sumit was mesmerised by the ocean when he laid eyes on it, soon after he arrived in Sydney as a boy.

'The first time I saw the ocean was in Christmas 1995,' recalls Sumit. 'I remember catching the 144 bus from Crows Nest to Manly Beach and gazing out at all this vast blue water that opened up in front of me when we came over the hill. I was just dazzled. In India, the equivalent is the Himalayas, but here it is the ocean.'

When Raaj moved to Sydney in her twenties, after their elaborate wedding in Punjab as part of their arranged marriage, Sumit was keen to show her the best of his home town. Sydney was certainly putting on her finest colours when Raaj arrived in late spring: the ocean was the colour of denim, the jasmine was blooming and there was the sound of currawongs around every corner.

She seems almost lost for words trying to describe the impact of the city's physical beauty. 'I kept looking up at the sky. It was so clear, so blue, so clean!' she says. 'And the water everywhere, in the harbour and at the beaches! To me it was, and still is, like living in paradise.'

The newlyweds began exploring Sydney: they went to the Opera House; they caught ferries; they bought board shorts and rashies and started splashing about in the local ocean pools and beaches. It was the first time Sumit had done so; he had spent much of his childhood sitting in the corner of the family restaurant doing his homework. He had little understanding of the sea around him. He'd watch other people dip in and out of the surf but he was afraid of the deep water, of losing balance, of losing control and drowning, and never ventured further than the shallows. In a swimming pool, he would hold on to the side or the steps with a vice-like grip.

He looks embarrassed when asked what finally prompted him to learn to swim. 'It was the end of the day, in summer, just after sunset,' he says slowly. 'The beach was unpatrolled. We both got in, but the next thing we knew, the waves were getting bigger and bigger.'

Neither Sumit nor Raaj was used to having water over their heads, let alone in a big surf. He watched Raaj's head disappear under a wave. Then another. To say it was terrifying is an understatement. He remembers the feeling of complete helplessness, and of gulping for air. He remembers calling out for help. He remembers holding his breath, as he held Raaj close. He remembers how quiet it all was, and the horrifying realisation that they would probably both drown without anyone around, without anyone seeing them.

But then, out of nowhere, they were saved by a good Samaritan, a lone surfer who saw they were in trouble, and paddled over.

'I remember every word he said, everything he did for us,' Sumit says, as he clears the table and orders tea. 'He had a strong, calm voice and just took control of the situation. He said to us, "Put your hands on my board. Hold on as tight as you can, and I'll take you back to the beach."

'When we got back to the shore, we were so shocked, and shaking. I remember looking up at the sky and feeling my feet on the ground and looking at this guy and just saying over and over and over again, "Thank you. Thank you. Thank you. Thank you."

'We were too young and foolish and shaken up to ask for his number or his name, but I will never forget his face. If he ever came forward we would so much love to show our appreciation. That guy saved our lives.'

Raaj and Sumit are not alone in underestimating the sea. On average, 288 people drown in Australia each year, and one in four of those are born overseas. The greatest numbers are among those born in India, Korea and Taiwan.

'After that night, we made a pact that we weren't going to tell anyone about it,' Sumit says. 'It put us both off swimming for years. We hardly even put a toe in the water, but now that we can swim, we like to tell people about it. We don't want anyone else making the same mistake we did.'

As destiny would have it, Raaj and Sumit found a gifted swimming teacher a few years later. Or rather, a teacher found them. When she heard about their near-drowning experience, Sue Bennett, a regular customer at their restaurant, offered to teach the couple in her own backyard pool for free.

Sue left the corporate world in 2014, and retrained as a coach with Swim Australia, prompted mainly by a story on the news about a migrant family whose child had drowned in South Sydney. She sits on the shoreline overlooking Collaroy Beach, radiating warmth and goodwill as she recounts that turning point. 'What an unimaginable situation. I was so shocked to think how those parents must have felt not being able to be safe enough themselves in the water to save their child. I knew then I wanted to teach adults to swim and share a love of the water.'

It seems like such an ordinary thing to many Australians – learning to swim. It's a way of life, something that usually starts before we attend school. Many of us spend so much

～～～

**Sumit was mesmerised by
the ocean when he laid eyes
on it, soon after he arrived
in Sydney as a boy.**

～～～

time in the water, and become so accustomed to swimming, that it's almost as easy, sometimes easier, than going for a walk.

But learning to swim as an adult is an entirely different matter. And teaching adults requires a different approach. 'When you're teaching babies and children,' Sue says, 'they just trust you instinctively. With adults you have to build trust first, before you can teach them to let go.'

Sumit was 36 and Raaj 28 when they finally turned up at Sue's home. She kitted them out with the tools of the trade – goggles, swim caps, kickboards – and then introduced them to the magic of buoyancy. In the first lesson they simply stood at the shallow end. She showed them how they could glide their hands through the water – and the beautiful quality of the liquid: that it moves around you, that you can push it and shape it around your body, but that it will also hold you.

'What I wanted to show them was that you can glide anywhere you like in water. You can float, and move to wherever you wish. There is zero gravity. And it's amazing.'

The next big breakthrough was teaching them to float. They lay on their backs, one at a time, and she stood right next to them, holding them from below. Each time they did it, she let go a little more, so that towards the end only her fingertips were gently touching their shoulders.

Whenever she saw them looking startled or their eyes grow wide with panic she would reassure them. 'I've got you,' she'd say. 'Look at me, you're safe. Breathe, stay calm, you've got this. I won't let anything happen to you.' It helps that she has the kind of soothing voice you could listen to all day. 'And remember, you're in the shallow end. If you want to, you can come out of the float and stand up.'

Sumit's take on learning to float? Nothing short of life-changing. 'We could feel her holding us, and we knew it was safe to let go, because she'd catch us if we started to sink. Learning to swim was exhilarating. First it was being able to relax enough to feel where you are in the water, in time and space, and how to get the sense of the water around you, and the pressure of it. Then, when we finally lifted our legs off the floor of the pool, and floated on our backs – no hands, no feet touching the floor or the side – and right over the deep end of her pool, well, that was …' he trails off, then after a long pause, adds, 'incredible.'

He shakes his head. 'To realise that if we were ever in an accident out at sea we could survive, if we just did that. All you have to do is float. I wish everyone knew how to do that.'

Under Sue's tutelage, Raaj and Sumit became competent swimmers, seemingly in no time. She led them step by step. First: walk to the other side of the pool. Second: put your face down, holding on to the side of the pool, and blow bubbles. She taught them how to breathe comfortably from either side. How to scull and tread water. And once they knew how to float, how to finally let go and glide from one side of the pool to the other. After that, it was time to circle their arms through the water and feel the power of doing freestyle.

All the while, she would distract them when they looked anxious. She'd just keep talking. Ask them about their plans for next weekend. Anything to cut through the fleeting thoughts of drowning.

Another of Sue's secrets in teaching adults is never to rush them, to let them learn at their own pace. She was amazed by the couple's determination. 'They turned up for lessons in the rain, and the wind, whatever the weather and season, whenever they got a break from their work.'

Within six weeks they felt safe enough to swim in the ocean pool and join the swimming fraternity that had been waiting just a few blocks from their busy restaurant.

'Everyone was always so encouraging when we'd come to swim at Collaroy pool,' Sumit recalls. 'They could see we were new to it, and kept telling us to keep coming. We felt like we'd joined a wonderful new club.'

Although both of them are still busy running the restaurant and looking after Kuwar, as well as holding down jobs in finance and IT, they look forward to joining a regular swim squad when their lives open up and they have more leisure time. They love the idea of gathering after ocean or pool swims for a coffee to discuss the swell, the bluebottles, the water temperature, the daily chitchat of their lives.

In a country like Australia, surrounded by the ocean, where so much of the population lives on the coast, knowing how to swim is something that truly matters, Sumit believes. 'I think for anyone coming to Australia, you should play a little video about important things you should and shouldn't do. And one of them is to swim between the flags. Australia is the most beautiful country, and I would say to anyone, come and enjoy it, but if you're going to stay here, you should learn how to swim. And pay attention to those red-and-yellow flags. If they're not up on the beach, don't go in.'

As for Raaj, the marine life at her doorstep calls and calls. Once she became confident swimming in Collaroy Rockpool, Sue taught her how to snorkel at Shelly Beach near the Cabbage Tree Bay Aquatic Reserve.

'I don't really have enough words to express what Sue has given me,' Raaj says. 'She opened up a new world for me, snorkelling at Shelly Beach. I didn't know you could see things like that. There are so many beautiful things under the water.' She's swum with cuttlefish, floated over a wobbegong, and gazed through her goggles at stingrays and once, a sea dragon. She's watched schools of wrasse swim through beds of sea grasses and, once or twice, come close enough to almost reach out and touch a blue groper.

It didn't take her long to buy a GoPro underwater camera. Before her mother died, in 2023, Raaj would send her footage of her swims. She was astonished by her daughter's new aquatic life.

Just like her husband, Raaj loves the camaraderie of local swimming groups, like the Bold and the Beautiful, who make their way from Manly to Shelly Beach every day, just after sunrise. The squad started with a small group of women

~~~

**Sumit's take on learning
to float? Nothing short of
life-changing.**

~~~

and has since grown to include hundreds of local ocean swimmers; their priority is staying safe, looking after each other and enjoying the ocean. Of less concern is the ability of the swimmer, or their cultural background.

For Raaj's first few swim attempts, Sue attached a waist strap with a swimming tow float as extra safety, and stayed right by her side as they completed the 1.2-kilometre swim together. They both left the beach that day streaming with salt water, feeling intensely alive. They did high fives on the shore, and vowed to do it again.

Raaj may not be able to get in the waves as much as she'd like right now, with their boisterous toddler underfoot, but she feels like she's learning a new language: getting to know how the currents move across the water, and to feel the pulse of the tides. She loves that just being near the ocean, and taking in great lungfuls of briny air, invigorates her, and heightens her senses. 'I'm just crazy about it, it's like a new love.'

In the meantime, Raaj and Sumit have become sponsors of the Collaroy Surf Life Saving Club. Kuwar is learning to swim and, when he's ready, they'll enrol him in Nippers, the local surf education program for children. Just like his parents, he adores the ocean. They call him their little fish.

CHAPTER 11

ERUB ARTS

Lost and Found

~~~

INSIDE THE TIMBER Erub Arts Centre in the Torres Strait, in the furthermost region of north-east Australia, Nancy Naawi is quietly humming a tune to herself. She is walking around a tablecloth-sized installation depicting the Great Barrier Reef. Nancy, who has lived in this small seafaring community all her life, has, with another artist, Florence Gutchen, spent weeks sewing, weaving and crocheting the piece from the offcuts of discarded fishing nets. She bends down over her work, pulling together the threads of bright pink, neon blue, orange and green, and pats her masterpiece proudly.

'There, it's done,' she says, walking out into the bright sunlight that pours into the art studio's courtyard. She sways a little, as if in private celebration.

Like most of the art made on Erub Island, about 200 kilometres north-east of Cape York, Nancy and Florence's work is far more than an ode to oceanic life. Look closer and you'll see that among the brilliantly hued stitching is a large white patch, representing coral bleaching. It's a stark warning about the environmental damage caused by ghost nets, which have been abandoned in South-East Asia and drift on strong ocean currents towards the far north Australian coast, and particularly the western regions of Torres Strait. Some of the nets have been cut loose from commercial fishing trawlers. Others are drift nets, many kilometres long, cast by fishers and left to float on the tides. Whatever the net, they all cut a swathe of destruction, indiscriminately trapping and killing marine life in their path.

Turtles make up the majority of the catch, but the nets also snare multitudes of other marine life: stingrays, coral trout, trevally, cuttlefish, dugongs, dolphins, sharks, jellyfish, octopus and squid. These invisible killing walls roll along the bottom of the ocean, entangling the coral of the nearby Great Barrier Reef as well as the mangroves lining the shores of the seventeen inhabited islands of the Torres Strait.

Instead of giving in to despair, the Erub Island artists have been tackling the problem head-on. Indigenous rangers – particularly those in the western islands of Torres Strait – have

It's a stark warning about the environmental damage caused by ghost nets.

been collecting the ocean refuse that washes up along the shores, hauling it onto barges and ships, and delivering it to the art centre for transformation.

The islands of the Torres Strait are scattered across the azure sea; as soon as you arrive on Erub (or Darnley) Island, you are enveloped in nature. It's the middle of June, and tropical storms have turned the roads to mud overnight. The ocean is choppy. Rough winds are still shaking the poinciana, bamboo and coconut palms, and scattering seabirds from the canopies into the sky. Despite the tumult, you can quickly see why this might be a Garden of Eden for the 400 Erub people who call this place home.

Inside the arts centre, it is a haven of tranquillity. A long wooden table is crammed with scissors, secateurs, net cutters, wire-cutters and baskets of ropes, nets and threads, as well as countless darning and sewing needles. Nancy, wearing a bright floral tunic and leather sandals, her tightly curled hair pulled back in a ponytail, sits beside two other artists, Lavinia Ketchell and Racy Oui-Pitt. The three women are head down, absorbed in making a series of turtles out of the deconstructed nets, comparing their needlework in a mixture of Creole and English.

'Does this look right?' Lavinia asks Racy. 'How did you get that stitching just right on the underside?'

Nancy and Racy, both elders of their community, take calls on their mobile phones from their grandchildren while a big metal urn simmers for morning tea. It would seem like your average craft group, if it weren't for the photos on the wall brightly cataloguing the Erub People's work.

Made in collaboration with non-Indigenous artists, the artworks are on display at such sites as the British Museum, the Le Havre Museum in France and the Oceanographic Museum in Monaco. Nancy points to a photo of one of the group's turtle installations on prominent display in the Musée d'ethnographie de Genève, in Switzerland. The 2-metre-long sea creature has an elaborately decorated shell, and is suspended from the ceiling of the prestigious institution. Another photo shows a hammerhead shark, acquired by the Asian Civilisations Museum in Singapore.

The meteoric rise of the Erub Art Centre's Ghost Net Project began in 2010, when Ghost Nets Australia, a federal government project, began collecting the increasingly alarming deposits of marine debris that washed up on our shores. Arts Queensland then funded a pilot project to bring non-Indigenous artists into First Nations groups to repurpose the fishing nets and ropes.

In these initial workshops, the group was encouraged to use these new materials in traditional crafting techniques to make small, practical objects such as bags, hats and cushions. As the group grew in confidence and size, it seemed only natural that the marine life they knew and loved would begin to emerge: colourful fish, frigatebirds, jellyfish, crocodiles, crayfish and dugongs. And turtles galore.

Their art blossomed at just the right time. With behind the scenes work by some of the group's non-Indigenous collaborators, who got the word out by networking with gallery owners and art collectors, the Erub artists were able to ride the wave of new-found global interest in ocean conservation.

The artists hit their stride in 2011, when they started making large installations; at the Cairns Indigenous Art Fair that year, a 2.5-metre squid called *Illum* caused a minor sensation.

Shortly afterwards, the Australian Museum in Sydney commissioned a 6-metre installation depicting a famous Erub Island love story between a giant rock cod and rock crab. Transported to Sydney in bubble wrap and wooden pallets, by barge, rail and truck, this artwork in particular, called *Dauma and Garom*, transfixes a steady stream of schoolchildren on excursion days as they troop through the museum's First Nations gallery. Then one of the Erub turtles, made by Ella Rose Savage, became an Australian stamp. The artists were putting Erub Island – one of the most remote parts of Australia – on the map, one stitch at a time.

There is an enormous amount of hard work involved in turning the sodden, filthy ropes and ghost nets into delicate sculptures. Many are picked up by marine debris clean-up boats from the Tangaroa Blue Foundation and the Australian Navy. Others are delivered to the island by the Sea Swift barge service.

Once on the island, the debris is hauled off the wharf in big bags by the rangers and taken by truck to the art studio. It's rough material to work with: salt encrusted and full of mud, barnacles, oysters and, often, the teeth of small fish that have been caught in the nets. It's all dragged to the back of the building, washed clean with a high-pressure hose, and then flung over the railings of the centre to dry in the sun.

After this forest of nets and ropes is untangled and sorted into colours, the artists get to work, stitching and stretching a first skin, or layer of netting, over the wire frames. On top of this, they add weaving, stitching, coils of fabric, embroidery, beads and shells.

Part of the secret of their success, many of them say, is the collaborative nature of their work. First Nations and non-Indigenous artists, such as Marion Gaemers, and the art centre's co-founders, Diann Lui and Lynnette Griffiths – all united in their love of the ocean – work side by side, sharing ideas and techniques to raise awareness of an increasingly alarming global problem. Often eight or nine artists will work on one piece at a time. 'We sit around talking about what we want to make,' Racy explains. 'We'll say, "Let's make the tail this big, and we'll cut the fins this way." We might make a big drawing in chalk on the cement in the courtyard of what we want to make, or on paper, and put it up on the wall, and we just start from there.' They also involve the local schoolchildren for some projects.

Lynnette, who got involved with Erub Arts when she was asked to facilitate one of the first workshops on the island, in 2010, often acted as a conduit between the Erub artists and the broader art world by being their unofficial sales manager. She had no hesitation in making cold calls to sell their work or using her contacts in the art world – or forging new ones. During her 20 years of involvement, Lynnette shared these skills with the Erub artists: how to put a value on their work when talking with dealers and collectors; how to overcome shyness. After the success of Erub, she wanted to expand the project, and set up the Ghost Net Collective, based in Cairns, which also creates art from abandoned beach debris.

One of the collective's best-known pieces is a series of brilliant illuminated giant rays, suspended from the ceiling of Sydney's Exchange Square in Barangaroo on the edge of Sydney Harbour. First Nations and non-Indigenous artists from all around the country – including Erub Island – contributed to the piece, crafting hundreds of tiny stingrays, which were then sewn into the underside of eleven 85-kilogram installations.

Making the ghost-net art is time-consuming, highly detailed business. The artists will spend months on each piece; the Barangaroo rays required eight months of stitching. It is soothing to watch them at work. They enjoy the creative process as much as the fruits of their labour. They chat, hum or sing as they work, listening to classic rock songs and sharing biscuits and cake. Every so often, they'll make each other cups of tea and share photos of weddings, parties and graduations. And then it's back to the craft.

'I like to work with ghost nets and ropes because it uses my fingers, my mind and my imagination,' Nancy explains.

Lavinia, listening in, agrees. 'It's nice being in your own headspace and using your imagination.'

A playful, lighthearted touch permeates their art. One fish sculpture is called Charles Boy. There is a jellyfish called Beryl, and a crocodile called Kenny. The Barangaroo stingrays? Why, they're Raynaldo, Raymond, Raynbow, Raylene and Raychel.

It's cultural practice on the island not to address relatives by their first names, so they call each other Ms Ketchell, Mrs Naawi and Mrs Pitt. But there is always time for a good joke. When Jimmy J. Thaiday, one of the best-known artists, walks in to join the women for a little while, no one respectfully calls him Mr Thaiday. 'Oh, everyone just calls him Gondo,' Racy teases.

Despite the laid-back atmosphere, though, the work is a deeply personal call to action, and a visceral reaction to the ocean damage – witnessed daily by the Erub people – caused by ghost nets and climate change.

'What people love about these artists is that they have created something beautiful out of a big, growing problem,' says Gladys Doolah, the art-centre manager. She's taking a break and sitting among the artists. 'The work comes from their heart. It is really important for them to tell their stories

~~~

The work is a deeply personal call to action, and a visceral reaction to the ocean damage.

~~~

about marine life – about how the ghost nets are ripping out the reef and all the marine animals are getting caught up in them – and people can pick that up.'

This makes so much sense. Erub Island is, after all, one of the few places in the world where the ocean is so embedded in everyday life that there are more boats than cars. Ferries and barges plough back and forth once a week between Erub and the administrative centre of Thursday Island, 200 kilometres away, delivering passengers, food and supplies. The main topic of conversation most days is the tides, the wind, the catch of the day and the best time to fish under the wharf.

The artists are all sea-life experts and care for animals deeply; they are so in tune with nature that they can recognise the particular subcategory of a fish by the shape of their eyes and mouths or the length of their tails. They can tell the sex of a turtle by the colour of its belly. The sea around Erub Island gives the artists a great sense of abundance. 'When we went to Sydney, I felt so sorry for the homeless people sleeping on the streets or in the railway stations,' Racy says, taking a needle out of her mouth to talk, her eyes glistening with tears. 'They look hungry. We get all our food free from the sea. We take as much as we need and nothing more.'

Every day, the islanders fish on the reef, either from a dinghy with a hand line or from the ancient stone fish traps lining the shore. 'The traps have been here so long, and we've been here so long, no one remembers how long they've been here for,' Racy says.

At lunchtime, one of the rangers goes down to check on the traps and demonstrates their ingenious design. In the morning, they remove some of the rocks making up part of the semicircular enclosure, as if opening a gate. By closing it an hour or two later, they can trap up to 200 fish a day.

There's no fast food on the island, and just one supermarket. Some of the islanders grow vegetables at home. Freshly caught mackerel, trevally and coral trout are mainstays in their diet. Racy loves to smoke or steam the fish, depending on her mood, or she'll make a fish stew out of lemongrass, ginger, garlic, onion and chilli paste. Fried octopus is a delicacy too, seasoned and cooked in banana leaves and coconut. On occasion there is fresh dugong, cooked underground for a long time in hot coals.

One of the mechanics from the mainland, 26-year-old Liam Bradley, working on the island on a three-week shift, says the seafood, caught on a hand line after work, is one of the perks of the job.

'I haven't had the chance to try turtle yet, but the other mechanics say if they had a choice between KFC and turtle, they'd take turtle every day,' he says, kicking off his workboots for the night. He's enjoying all the other local seafood in the meantime. 'The squid! Soak it overnight in milk, then flour it and fry it: it's fuckin awesome. Nothing like it.'

The relationship between island life and its environment is a delicate one. Many of the locals have witnessed dramatic coral bleaching in the nearby Great Barrier Reef, and have been alarmed by the sight of sardine shoals lying stranded on the beach during marine heatwaves. Rising sea levels threaten the gentle rhythms of the ecosystem. 'I feel sorry for the birds,' Nancy says. 'They've got nowhere to nest. The grass where they used to nest has been covered by water. Where are they going to go now?' She has been busy working this whole time, weaving the thread through and over. 'When I see the coral dying, I feel like I have to do something about it.' She gestures to the netting on their worktable. 'This is my way of telling people what's going on. I grew up swimming, diving and fishing here and it makes me sad to see what the ghost nets are doing to our creatures.'

Beside her, Racy shakes her head. 'I often feel emotional when I am making our pieces. When you see the whales, how magnificent and graceful they are, it just makes you feel so good to be alive.'

What does she think about as she weaves? She pauses, looks suddenly serious. 'I hope they might make people more aware of what to do with their nets. Think about marine life before you just leave them there in the ocean. Do something about it. We always cry a little bit when we've finished a big piece, because we put so much work into them,' she says. 'It's hard to let go of them because they are so personal.'

Helping to heal the ocean, by shining a light on the problem of ocean debris, is a reciprocal act. For many of the Erub artists, particularly the older women, the ocean has helped them forge a new career, and carve out recognition for themselves and their community. Racy was almost pinching herself when she first laid eyes on the stingrays suspended from the Exchange Square ceiling. 'We were so happy to see them up there. When you look up, it feels like being on the ocean floor looking up at the reflections.'

The rays have a special meaning for her; they were inspired by her memories of boat trips to Thursday Island and the mainland, long before there were plane and ferry services to Erub. 'We'd stay in the boat at night, and we always loved the colours of the stars reflected on the sea. The sea looks incredibly beautiful by moonlight.'

Staging their exhibitions has also given the artists the opportunity to travel. Lavinia lists the places she's been to: Singapore, Monaco, Cambridge, Canada, New Caledonia, Washington, Charlottesville, New York, Darwin, Alice Springs, Perth and Uluru. 'How many people have had the chance to do that?' she asks.

As part of the exhibitions, the artists usually give talks at art workshops. The challenge, they find, is expressing what they really mean in English, rather than Creole, their first language. Nancy, helping herself to a biscuit, laughs infectiously. 'Speaking English too much makes my mouth hurt.'

~~~

'I grew up swimming, diving and fishing here, and it makes me sad to see what the ghost nets are doing to our creatures.'

~~~

Although money-making is usually the furthest thing from their minds, the people of Erub Arts head a well-run business. The most expensive artwork was a large turtle, sold for $65,000; the smaller works sell for around $1200. Social media helps with sales too. During the first lockdown in 2020, when the COVID-19 pandemic arrived, Lynnette designed kits to make turtles and fish at home. They sold out within 20 minutes of a Facebook post going live.

Fame and fanfare are of little interest to most of the artists. You could hardly tell from his unassuming manner, but Jimmy is a highly accomplished artist whose work is on display at the Australian Museum and the National Gallery of Victoria. He likes living quietly – fishing, diving and walking on the reef – but he has a keen sense of purpose, and this beams through. Like most islanders, his knowledge of its creatures and seasons is intimate.

'We are saltwater people,' he says, holding up a large sculpture of a frigatebird he is working on. He imitates the action of flying. 'They are weathervanes,' he explains. 'If they are flying high, it means the winds will stop in the next day, and the weather will be fine. If they are flying low, it means it will be very windy in the next day. They're like pirates of the air – they'll swoop down and steal fish out of the beaks of other birds.'

He's also drawn to the hammerhead sharks that are often seen on the north-west side of the reef. They have inspired several magnificent sculptures he and his brother have created. 'They swim up from the deep water to feast. They're really, really smart.'

He winces when asked about the damage caused by the ghost nets. 'The ghost nets are choking the trees, as well as killing the turtles and sharks and manta rays and big eagle rays – it's a terrible thing to see them caught like that.'

When it comes to the commercial fishing trawlers, he folds his arms in weary acceptance. 'It's all about the money to them – they cut off the big nets from their boats and let them go out to sea because they can't be bothered to pull them in and clean up after themselves. They've got dollar signs in their eyes. If they fished the way Traditional Owners fished – only taking what they needed – there would be no problem, no pollution.'

Jimmy walks upstairs to the art centre gift shop. Each of the centre's three octagonal-shaped buildings was architecturally designed to echo the traditional beehive hut built on the island before first contact. He flips over the large stand that displays many of their screen-prints. Most of the designs are inspired by the artists' childhoods or the stories of their ancestors, and the demand for them remains strong. One of the most popular is the trochus shells. 'We would all dive for them, clean them, eat the meat out of it, or use it for bait, or sell the meat ... or shells.'

He points to another popular one: a striking black-and-white print of the heavy metal helmets used by Japanese divers off the island in the 1920s and 1930s. Jimmy's parents and grandparents told him about the divers: they were usually young men, often from the poorer districts of Japan, and they would dive to treacherously deep levels – sometimes up to 20 metres – to collect lucrative mother-of-pearl shells before plastic buttons flooded the market.

'When the basket was full, they would pull on the rope to bring them up from the bottom of the ocean,' Jimmy explains. 'It was dangerous work, they didn't get paid much, and there were signs of people in town with the bends.' (The shaking caused by decompression sickness from rising to the surface too quickly.) There are graveyards on all the islands of the Torres Strait honouring the many Indigenous and Japanese divers who lost their lives in 'the Darnley Deep', the sea around Erub Island.

All around the centre, suspended from the ceiling and stacked on the shelves, are sculptures ready for the upcoming Indigenous art fairs in Cairns and Darwin. Wandering beneath and among them feels like plunging into a dream world under the waves. Some of the faces of the fish and rays are so friendly that they look like they might speak. It's no surprise that children adore them, instinctively reaching out to touch them.

Being up close with these giant stingrays and turtles – even the large sharks – prompts a new view of marine life, with fresh eyes: with curiosity and respect rather than fear. And, more than anything else, they allow us to see clearly how much is at stake.

'All these good things come from the sea,' Jimmy says as he packs away his wire-cutters and baskets of ropes and nets for the night. 'Why would you want to do anything to destroy it?'

Acknowledgements

THIS BOOK WOULD not have been possible without my partner, Bryce, who cheerfully drove me several thousand kilometres along the coastline of New South Wales, bundled me onto long distance trains, and arranged for me – after much reassurance – to catch several extremely small planes to interview the subjects of this book. His absence of doubt is a large part of its success.

I am indebted to publisher Alexandra Payne at Murdoch Books and literary agent Lyn Tranter; they immediately saw the value of these stories and shared in the contagious zest of their creation. It was my good fortune to work with editor Emma Schwarcz, who meticulously beat each chapter into shape.

To Claire Vince at The Australian Museum – your part in introducing me to Jessica Watson, Valerie Taylor, Dr Chels Marshall and the Erub artists is gratefully acknowledged.

To my family – my gratitude, as always, for your incredible generosity. A special thanks goes to my dearest mates Julie and Lou, for their ability to make me laugh until I cry, for their wisdom, and for always being by my side. Praise is also due to writer Sue Williams and journalist Wally Mason for their sterling advice.

Lastly, my sincere thanks to the people in this book, all united in their love of the ocean, who welcomed me into their homes, studios, local cafés, beaches, rock pools and favourite bodies of salt water, and who so generously shared their time and thoughts. It was an honour to be entrusted with your stories.

Resources

~~~

Australian Marine Conservation Society:
  marineconservation.org.au
Autism Swim: **autisumswim.com.au**
Boardriders clubs: **surfingaustralia.com/clubs**
Dippers: **autismswim.com.au/dippers**
Erub Arts: **erubarts.com.au**
The Fred Hollows Foundation: **hollows.org**
Ghost Nets Australia:
  parksaustralia.gov.au/ghost-nets-initiative
National Parks and Wildlife Service:
  nationalparks.nsw.gov.au
Rainbow Club: **rainbowclub.au**
Swim Sisters: **instagram.com/swimsisterssquad**
Surf Life Saving Australia: **sls.com.au**
Tangaroa Blue: **tangaroablue.org**
Veteran Surf Project: **veteransurfproject.org**

About the Interviewees

~~~

Chloe Alder has a strong sense of social justice and is a fierce advocate for inclusion, particularly in her role as Operations Manager with Autism Swim. With two boys on the spectrum and a neurotypical daughter, she leads a very busy life but enjoys taking time out at the beach with her children on the weekends.

~~~

Layne Beachley (AO) is a renowned Australian surfer with seven World Championship titles. She has been a tireless advocate for women's surfing and, in 2003, founded the Layne Beachley Aim for the Stars Foundation. She has been inducted into the Australian Surfing Hall of Fame and was appointed an Officer of the Order of Australia in 2015.

Erub Arts Centre is located on Erub (Darnley) Island in Torres Strait. Dedicated to preserving and promoting the artistic heritage of the Torres Strait Islander people, the Erub Arts fosters cultural expression and creativity, offers a space for artists to work, runs workshops, exhibitions and cultural programs, and collaborates with cultural institutions, galleries and organisations to showcase the work of its artists.

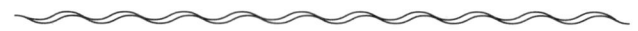

Erika Gleeson (GC Autism Studies, BA Behavioural Science) is a Senior Behaviour Specialist, having spent the past sixteen years enhancing the lives of those with a disability. She is founder of the award-winning charity Autism Swim, an international organisation aimed at making aquatics inclusive. Erika is a renowned speaker, author and finalist for Australian of the Year (2021).

Rajbir Kaur (Raaj) was born in India and, after an arranged marriage to Sumit, she migrated to Australia at 24. As well as raising their son, Kuwar, and supporting the family restaurant, GurTaj, Raaj is a CRM system analyst for a leading payroll software company. She swims with the Bold and Beautiful swim squad at Manly, and enjoys making chilli oil from scorpion chillies and garlic from her own backyard.

Dr Chels Marshall is a leading Indigenous marine scientist. A Gumbaynggirr woman from Valla on the Mid North Coast of New South Wales, she is renowned for integrating Aboriginal ecological knowledge with contemporary environmental practices and design, and is an advocate for sustainable development and cultural preservation.

Yusra Metwally is an Egyptian–Australian solicitor working with victim–survivors of domestic violence. She is also a community advocate, a writer and the founder of Swim Sisters, a grassroots initiative promoting inclusivity in swimming for Muslim and culturally diverse women. With a policy background, Yusra is dedicated to amplifying marginalised voices and bridging the gap between policy and practice.

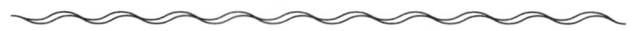

Rusty Moran is a PhD candidate at Western Sydney University studying surf therapy as a treatment for veterans with PTSD, and is the founder of Veteran Surf Project, a charity helping veterans and first responders. A former professional surfer, Rusty operates a surf school catering for children and adults with disabilities.

Tony Pearce joined the army as a seventeen-year-old and, after being discharged due to PTSD, spent the next twenty years lost in addiction, ultimately losing everything and everyone important in his life. At 51, his life finally changed when he found the Veteran Surf Project and the ocean.

James Pittar is an Australian marathon swimmer. He was the first Australian to complete the Triple Crown of Open Water Swimming – the English Channel, the Manhattan Island Marathon and the Catalina Channel. In the process, he became the first blind person to complete each event.

Derek Pyrah was diagnosed with PTSD following service in Iraq, was prescribed psychiatric medications for more than seventeen years and subsequently suffered great loss. He stabilised and started rebuilding his life with medicinal cannabis and by connecting to the ocean through surfing. Derek is fighting for Veterans Affairs to re-approve medicinal cannabis for PTSD veterans.

Sumit Singh is client relations manager, responsible for shareholder management for listed ASX companies. Sumit also supports his family's popular Indian restaurant, GurTaj, in Collaroy on the Northern Beaches. The business is proactive in supporting local community initiatives by supporting local clubs and hosting events. GurTaj was one of the first local businesses to offer free food during the COVID lockdowns.

Valerie Taylor (AM) is an Australian marine conservationist, filmmaker and photographer who has collaborated on iconic documentaries and films, including *Jaws*. She has received numerous honours, including being made a Member of the Order of Australia and being inducted into the International Scuba Diving Hall of Fame. Valerie was knighted by the Dutch Royal family for her successful work in the field of marine conservation. She is currently an ambassador for the Sydney Institute of Marine Science.

Jessica Watson (OAM) navigated some of the world's most remote oceans and survived 210 days alone at sea at age sixteen to become the youngest person to sail nonstop around the world solo. She was named Young Australian of the Year in 2011. Now 31, Jessica has completed an MBA, and authored two books, the best-selling memoir *True Spirit* and the middle-grade novel *Indigo Blue*. She is a management consultant in Deloitte's Human Capital consulting team.

Tim Winton (AO) is the author of 30 books for adults and children. Among many accolades are his four Miles Franklin Literary Awards (for *Shallows*, *Cloudstreet*, *Dirt Music* and *Breath*). His work has been translated into many languages, and adapted for stage, film, television and radio.